FDG PET/CT Imaging: Normal Variations and Benign Findings

Editors

MOHSEN BEHESHTI
CHUN K. KIM

PET CLINICS

www.pet.theclinics.com

Consulting Editor
ABASS ALAVI

April 2014 • Volume 9 • Number 2

ELSEVIER

1600 John F. Kennedy Boulevard • Suite 1800 • Philadelphia, Pennsylvania, 19103-2899

http://www.theclinics.com

PET CLINICS Volume 9, Number 2
April 2014 ISSN 1556-8598, ISBN-13: 978-0-323-29008-1

Publisher: John Vassallo
Developmental Editor: Susan Showalter

PET Clinics (ISSN 1556-8598) is published quarterly by Elsevier Inc., 360 Park Avenue South, New York, NY 10010-1710. Months of issue are January, April, July, and October. Periodicals postage paid at New York, NY, and additional mailing offices. Subscription prices per year are $225.00 (US individuals), $327.00 (US institutions), $115.00 (US students), $255.00 (Canadian individuals), $369.00 (Canadian institutions), $140.00 (Canadian students), $275.00 (foreign individuals), $369.00 (foreign institutions), and $140.00 (foreign students). To receive student and resident rate, orders must be accompanied by name of affiliated institution, date of term, and the signature of program/residency coordinator on institution letterhead. Orders will be billed at individual rate until proof of status is received. Foreign air speed delivery is included in all Clinics subscription prices. All prices are subject to change without notice. POSTMASTER: Send address changes to PET Clinics, Elsevier Health Sciences Division, Subscription Customer Service, 3251 Riverport Lane, Maryland Heights, MO 63043. **Customer Service: 1-800-654-2452 (U.S. and Canada); 314-447-8871 (outside U.S. and Canada). Fax: 314-447-8029. E-mail: journalscustomerservice-usa@elsevier.com (for print support); journalsonlinesupport-usa@elsevier.com (for online support).**

Reprints. For copies of 100 or more of articles in this publication, please contact the Commercial Reprints Department, Elsevier Inc., 360 Park Avenue South, New York, NY 10010-1710. Tel.: 212-633-3874; Fax: 212-633-3820; E-mail: reprints@elsevier.com.

Printed and bound by CPI Group (UK) Ltd, Croydon, CR0 4YY

Contributors

CONSULTING EDITOR

ABASS ALAVI, MD (Hon), PhD (Hon), DSc (Hon)
Professor of Radiology, Division of Nuclear Medicine, Department of Radiology, University of Pennsylvania School of Medicine, Hospital of the University of Pennsylvania, Pennsylvania University, Philadelphia, Pennsylvania

EDITORS

MOHSEN BEHESHTI, MD, FASNC, FEBNM
Head, PET-CT Center LINZ, Associate Professor in Nuclear Medicine, Department of Nuclear Medicine and Endocrinology, St. Vincent's Hospital, Linz, Austria

CHUN K. KIM, MD
Associate Professor of Radiology, Harvard Medical School; Clinical Director, Division of Nuclear Medicine and Molecular Imaging, Brigham and Women's Hospital, Boston, Massachusetts

AUTHORS

SCOTT R. AKERS, MD, PhD
Department of Radiology, Philadelphia VA Medical Center, Philadelphia, Pennsylvania

ABASS ALAVI, MD (Hon), PhD (Hon), DSc (Hon)
Professor of Radiology, Division of Nuclear Medicine, Department of Radiology, University of Pennsylvania School of Medicine, Hospital of the University of Pennsylvania, Pennsylvania University, Philadelphia, Pennsylvania

NORBERT E. AVRIL, MD
Department of Radiology, Case Western Reserve University, University Hospitals Case Medical Center, Cleveland, Ohio

LUIS S. BELTRAN, MD
Department of Radiology, New York University School of Medicine, New York, New York

ANNE KIIL BERTHELSEN, MD
Department of Clinical Physiology, Nuclear Medicine and PET, Rigshospitalet, University of Copenhagen, Copenhagen, Denmark

VALENTINA BERTI, MD, PhD
Nuclear Medicine Unit, Department of Biomedical, Experimental and Clinical Sciences, University of Florence, Florence, Italy

HERSH CHANDARANA, MD
Department of Radiology, New York University School of Medicine, New York, New York

GANG CHENG, MD, PhD
Department of Radiology, Philadelphia VA Medical Center; Department of Radiology, Hospital of the University of Pennsylvania, Philadelphia, Pennsylvania

LIRAN DOMACHEVSKY, MD
Department of Imaging, Dana-Farber Cancer Institute; Division of Nuclear Medicine and Molecular Imaging, Department of Radiology, Brigham and Women's Hospital; Assistant Professor, Harvard Medical School, Boston, Massachusetts

KENT P. FRIEDMAN, MD
Department of Radiology, New York University
School of Medicine, New York, New York

CRISTINA GÁMEZ-CENZANO, MD, PhD
Director, PET-Unit, Institut de Diagnòstic per la
Imatge (IDI), Hospital Universitari de Bellvitge–
IDIBELL, L'Hospitalet de Llobregat, Barcelona,
Spain

CHRISTIAN GEPPERT, PhD
MR R&D Collaborations, Siemens Healthcare,
New York, New York

VICTOR H. GERBAUDO, PhD, MSHCA
Director, Nuclear Medicine and Molecular
Imaging Program, Associate Director, Center
for Pulmonary Functional Imaging (Oncology),
Associate Scientific Director, Advanced
Multimodality Image Guided Operating
Suite, Assistant Professor of Radiology,
Harvard Medical School, Boston,
Massachusetts

FREDERICK D. GRANT, MD
Division of Nuclear Medicine and Molecular
Imaging, Department of Radiology, Boston
Children's Hospital; Assistant Professor in
Radiology, Harvard Medical School;
Training Program Director, Harvard Joint
Program in Nuclear Medicine, Boston,
Massachusetts

LISELOTTE HØJGAARD, MD, DMSCi
Professor, Department of Clinical Physiology,
Nuclear Medicine and PET, Faculty of Health
and Medical Sciences, Rigshospitalet, University
of Copenhagen, Copenhagen, Denmark

HEATHER A. JACENE, MD
Clinical Director, Department of Imaging,
Dana-Farber Cancer Institute; Division of
Nuclear Medicine and Molecular Imaging,
Department of Radiology, Brigham and
Women's Hospital; Associate Professor,
Harvard Medical School, Boston,
Massachusetts

CHUN K. KIM, MD
Associate Professor of Radiology, Harvard
Medical School; Clinical Director, Division of
Nuclear Medicine and Molecular Imaging,
Brigham and Women's Hospital, Boston,
Massachusetts

ANDRES KOHAN, MD
Department of Radiology, Case Western
Reserve University, University Hospitals
Case Medical Center, Cleveland, Ohio;
Department of Radiology, Hospital Italiano de
Buenos Aires, Ciudad Autónoma de Buenos
Aires, Argentina

NAM JU LEE, MD
Department of Radiology, Hospital of the
University of Pennsylvania, Philadelphia,
Pennsylvania

ANNIKA LOFT, MD, PhD
Department of Clinical Physiology,
Nuclear Medicine and PET, Rigshospitalet,
University of Copenhagen, Copenhagen,
Denmark

LISA MOSCONI, PhD
Center for Brain Health, New York
University School of Medicine, New York,
New York

FRANCISCO PINO-SORROCHE, PhD
Physicist, Medical Physics Department, Institut
Català d'Oncologia (ICO), Hospital Duran i
Reynals–IDIBELL, L'Hospitalet de Llobregat,
Barcelona, Spain

FABIO PONZO, MD
Department of Radiology, New York
University School of Medicine, New York,
New York

ALBERTO PUPI, MD
Nuclear Medicine Unit, Department of
Biomedical, Experimental and Clinical
Sciences, University of Florence, Florence,
Italy

RAJAN RAKHEJA, MD
Clinical Assistant Professor of Medical
Imaging, Department of Nuclear Medicine/
Radiology, Royal University Hospital,
Saskatoon, Saskatchewan, Canada

CHRISTOPHER G. SAKELLIS, MD
Department of Imaging, Dana-Farber Cancer
Institute; Division of Nuclear Medicine and
Molecular Imaging, Department of Radiology,
Brigham and Women's Hospital; Instructor,
Harvard Medical School, Boston,
Massachusetts

ALEXANDRA L. SELTZER, MD
Department of Radiology, New York University
School of Medicine, New York, New York

JASON W. WACHSMANN, MD
Fellow, Joint Program in Nuclear Medicine,
Division of Nuclear Medicine and Molecular
Imaging, Department of Radiology, Brigham
and Women's Hospital, Harvard Medical
School, Boston, Massachusetts

KATHERINE ZUKOTYNSKI, MD
Staff Radiologist and Assistant Professor,
Department of Medical Imaging,
Sunnybrook Health Sciences Centre,
University of Toronto, Ontario, Canada;
Research Associate and Visiting Assistant
Professor, Department of Radiology,
Brigham and Women's Hospital,
Harvard Medical School, Boston,
Massachusetts

ALEXANDRA L. SELTZER, MD
Department of Radiology, New York University
School of Medicine, New York, New York

JASON W. WACHSMANN, MD
Fellow, Joint Program in Nuclear Medicine,
Division of Nuclear Medicine and Molecular
Imaging, Department of Radiology, Brigham
and Women's Hospital, Harvard Medical
School, Boston, Massachusetts

KATHERINE ZUKOTYNSKI, MD
Staff Radiologist and Assistant Professor,
Department of Medical Imaging,
Sunnybrook Health Sciences Centre,
University of Toronto, Ontario, Canada;
Research Associate and Visiting Assistant
Professor, Department of Radiology,
Brigham and Women's Hospital,
Harvard Medical School, Boston,
Massachusetts

Contents

Preface: FDG PET/CT: Normal Variations and Benign Findings - Translation to PET/MRI   xiii

Mohsen Beheshti and Chun K. Kim

Standardization and Quantification in FDG-PET/CT Imaging for Staging and Restaging of Malignant Disease   117

Cristina Gámez-Cenzano and Francisco Pino-Sorroche

There is a growing interest in using quantification in FDG-PET/CT in oncology, especially for evaluating response to therapy. Complex full quantitative procedures with blood sampling and dynamic scanning have been clinically replaced by the use of standardized uptake value measurements that provide an index of regional tracer uptake normalized to the administered dose of FDG. Some approaches have been proposed for assessing quantitative metabolic response, such as EORTC and PERCIST criteria in solid tumors. When using standardized uptake value in clinical routine and multicenter trials, standardization of protocols and quality control procedures of instrumentation is required.

Brain: Normal Variations and Benign Findings in Fluorodeoxyglucose-PET/Computed Tomography Imaging   129

Valentina Berti, Lisa Mosconi, and Alberto Pupi

Brain 18F-fluorodeoxyglucose (18F-FDG) PET allows the in vivo study of cerebral glucose metabolism, reflecting neuronal and synaptic activity. 18F-FDG-PET has been extensively used to detect metabolic alterations in several neurologic diseases compared with normal aging. However, healthy subjects have variants of 18F-FDG distribution, especially as associated with aging. This article focuses on 18F-FDG-PET findings in so-called normal brain aging, and in particular on metabolic differences occurring with aging and as a function of people's gender. The effect of different substances, medications, and therapy procedures are discussed, as well as common artifacts.

Head and Neck: Normal Variations and Benign Findings in FDG Positron Emission Tomography/Computed Tomography Imaging   141

Liselotte Højgaard, Anne Kiil Berthelsen, and Annika Loft

Positron emission tomography (PET)/computed tomography with FDG of the head and neck region is mainly used for the diagnosis of head and neck cancer, for staging, treatment evaluation, relapse, and planning of surgery and radio therapy. This article is a practical guide of imaging techniques, including a detailed protocol for FDG PET in head and neck imaging, physiologic findings, and pitfalls in selected case stories.

Thorax: Normal and Benign Pathologic Patterns in FDG-PET/CT Imaging   147

Jason W. Wachsmann and Victor H. Gerbaudo

This article describes the normal patterns of thoracic 18F-fluorodeoxyglucose (FDG) biodistribution, and expands on the role of FDG-PET/computed tomography (CT) for the evaluation of patients suffering from a spectrum of benign pathologic conditions that affect the chest. The discussion addresses the applications of FDG-PET/CT imaging in a wide variety of chest-related disorders. Familiarity with the normal thoracic biodistribution of FDG, coupled with knowledge of the potential nonmalignant causes of increased FDG uptake in the chest, is essential to minimize the incidence of incorrect interpretation of FDG-PET images in daily clinical practice.

Abdomen: Normal Variations and Benign Conditions Resulting in Uptake on FDG-PET/CT

169

Katherine Zukotynski and Chun K. Kim

The increasing use of ^{18}F-fluorodeoxyglucose positron emission tomography/computed tomography (FDG-PET/CT) in oncology has led to: improved sensitivity and specificity in detecting localized and metastatic disease, increased ability to target biopsies to the site of most aggressive disease, and development of a noninvasive biomarker to assess prognosis and effects of therapy. However, for correct interpretation of FDG-PET/CT studies, an understanding of both normal and abnormal imaging appearances commonly encountered in oncology patients is important. This article discusses commonly seen normal variations and benign findings on FDG-PET/CT of the abdomen.

Pelvis: Normal Variants and Benign Findings in FDG-PET/CT Imaging

185

Andres Kohan and Norbert E. Avril

With the widespread use of whole-body fluorodeoxyglucose (FDG)-PET/computed tomography as a diagnostic tool in patients with cancer, incidental findings are of increasing importance. This is particularly true within the pelvis, where several benign findings might present with increased FDG uptake. In addition, physiologic excretion of radiotracer by way of the urinary tract can complicate image analysis. This article reviews potential incidental benign findings in the pelvis that one should be aware of when interpreting FDG-PET/computed tomography scans.

Normal Variations and Benign Findings in Pediatric ^{18}F-FDG-PET/CT

195

Frederick D. Grant

^{18}F-FDG PET and PET/CT have a wide variety of indications in children and young adults. Oncologic indications are the most common, but others include neurology, sports medicine, cardiology, and infection imaging. Accurate interpretation of pediatric ^{18}F-FDG PET and PET/CT requires a technically adequate study and knowledgeable interpretation of the images. A successful pediatric ^{18}F-FDG PET requires age-appropriate patient preparation and consideration of patient age and developmental stage. Accurate interpretation of the study requires familiarity with normal patterns of physiologic ^{18}F-FDG uptake in children at all stages of development.

Differential Background Clearance of Fluorodeoxyglucose Activity in Normal Tissues and its Clinical Significance

209

Gang Cheng, Abass Alavi, Nam Ju Lee, and Scott R. Akers

The clearance of 2-deoxy-2-[18F]fluoro-D-glucose (FDG) activity in normal tissues varies significantly with extended distribution time. Although most tissues have lower standardized uptake value (SUV) on 2-hour/3-hour delayed images, others may have stable or higher FDG activity with longer distribution times. The continuously decreased SUV on delayed imaging in some tissues, especially in the liver, indicates that longer distribution time will decrease background activity, increase lesion-to-background ratio, and thus improve imaging quality, whereas the continuously increased SUV from 1 to 3 hours in the heart suggest that longer distribution time will improve detection of viable myocardium in a viability study.

Postradiation Changes in Tissues: Evaluation by Imaging Studies with Emphasis on Fluorodeoxyglucose-PET/Computed Tomography and Correlation with Histopathologic Findings   **217**

Liran Domachevsky, Heather A. Jacene, Christopher G. Sakellis, and Chun K. Kim

Efforts have been made to minimize the damage to adjacent normal tissues during radiotherapy, primarily by shifting from the use of conventional radiotherapy to more advanced techniques. Reviewing the overall pattern on combined anatomic and functional imaging can enhance diagnostic accuracy. Several radiotracers can be used; [18F]fluorodeoxyglucose is the most common. Familiarity with the type and timing of previous radiation therapy, the spectrum of imaging findings after radiation injury, and the appropriate use of the different radiotracers can be crucial. This article summarizes postradiation histologic findings and multimodality imaging findings, with emphasis on PET/computed tomography.

Fluorodeoxyglucose Positron Emission Tomography/Magnetic Resonance Imaging: Current Status, Future Aspects   **237**

Rajan Rakheja, Hersh Chandarana, Fabio Ponzo, Alexandra L. Seltzer, Luis S. Beltran, Christian Geppert, and Kent P. Friedman

Simultaneous positron emission tomography (PET)/magnetic resonance (MR) imaging is a promising novel technology for oncology diagnosis and staging and neurologic and cardiac applications. Our institution's current research protocol results in a total imaging time of approximately 45 to 70 minutes with simultaneous PET/MR imaging, making this a feasible total body imaging protocol. Further development of MR-based attenuation correction will improve PET quantification. Quantitatively accurate multiparametric PET/MR data sets will likely improve diagnosis of disease and help guide and monitor the therapies for individualized patient care.

Index   **253**

PET CLINICS

FORTHCOMING ISSUES

July 2014
PET/CT Imaging in Tracers Beyond FDG
Mohsen Beheshti and Chun K. Kim, *Editors*

October 2014
Contributions of FDG to Modern Medicine, Part I
Søren Hess and Poul Flemming Høilund-Carlsen, *Editors*

January 2015
Clinical Applications of FDG, Part II
Søren Hess and Poul Flemming Høilund-Carlsen, *Editors*

RECENT ISSUES

January 2014
Management of Neuroendocrine Tumors
Stefano Fanti, Cristina Nanni, and Richard Baum, *Editors*

October 2013
Novel Imaging Techniques in Neurodegenerative and Movement Disorders
Rathan M. Subramaniam and Jorge R. Barrio, *Editors*

July 2013
Evolving Medical Imaging Techniques
Thomas C. Kwee and Habib Zaidi, *Editors*

PROGRAM OBJECTIVE

The goal of the PET Clinics is to keep practicing radiologists and radiology residents up to date with current clinical practice in positron emission tomography by providing timely articles reviewing the state of the art in patient care.

TARGET AUDIENCE

Practicing radiologists, radiology residents, and other health care professionals who provide patient care utilizing radiologic findings.

LEARNING OBJECTIVES

Upon completion of this activity, participants will be able to:

1. Review standardization and quantification in FDG-PET/CT imaging for staging and restaging of malignant disease.
2. Discuss the current status and future aspects of FDG PET/MRI.
3. Recognize normal and benign pathologic patterns in FDG-PET/CT imaging of the pelvis, thorax, brain, abdomen, and the head and neck.

ACCREDITATION

The Elsevier Office of Continuing Medical Education (EOCME) is accredited by the Accreditation Council for Continuing Medical Education (ACCME) to provide continuing medical education for physicians.

The EOCME designates this enduring material for a maximum of 15 *AMA PRA Category 1 Credit*(s)™. Physicians should claim only the credit commensurate with the extent of their participation in the activity.

All other health care professionals requesting continuing education credit for this enduring material will be issued a certificate of participation.

DISCLOSURE OF CONFLICTS OF INTEREST

The EOCME assesses conflict of interest with its instructors, faculty, planners, and other individuals who are in a position to control the content of CME activities. All relevant conflicts of interest that are identified are thoroughly vetted by EOCME for fair balance, scientific objectivity, and patient care recommendations. EOCME is committed to providing its learners with CME activities that promote improvements or quality in healthcare and not a specific proprietary business or a commercial interest.

The planning committee, staff, authors and editors listed below have identified no financial relationships or relationships to products or devices they or their spouse/life partner have with commercial interest related to the content of this CME activity:

Scott R. Akers, MD, PhD; Abass Alavi, MD; Norbert E. Avril, MD; Mohsen Beheshti, MD; Luis S. Beltran, MD; Anne Kiil Berthelsen, MD; Valentina Berti, MD, PhD; Adrianne Brigido; Hersh Chandarana, MD; Gang Cheng, MD, PhD; Liran Domachevsky, MD; Kent P. Friedman, MD; Cristina Gámez-Cenzano, MD, PhD; Victor H. Gerbaudo, PhD, MSHCA; Frederick D. Grant, MD; Kristen Helm; Liselotte Højgaard, MD, DMSci; Brynne Hunter; Heather A. Jacene, MD; Chun K. Kim, MD; Andres Kohan, MD; Nam Ju Lee, MD; Annika Loft, MD, PhD; Sandy Lavery; Jill McNair; Lisa Mosconi, PhD; Mahalakshmi Narayanan; Francisco Pino-Sorroche, PhD; Fabio Ponzo, MD; Alberto Pupi, MD; Rajan Rakheja, MD; Christopher G. Sakellis, MD; Alexandra L. Seltzer, MD; Jason W. Wachsmann, MD; Katherine Zukotynski, MD.

The planning committee, staff, authors and editors listed below have identified financial relationships or relationships to products or devices they or their spouse/life partner have with commercial interest related to the content of this CME activity:

Christian Geppert, PhD has an employment affiliation with Siemens AG.

UNAPPROVED/OFF-LABEL USE DISCLOSURE

The EOCME requires CME faculty to disclose to the participants:

1. When products or procedures being discussed are off-label, unlabelled, experimental, and/or investigational (not US Food and Drug Administration (FDA) approved); and
2. Any limitations on the information presented, such as data that are preliminary or that represent ongoing research, interim analyses, and/or unsupported opinions. Faculty may discuss information about pharmaceutical agents that is outside of FDA-approved labelling. This information is intended solely for CME and is not intended to promote off-label use of these medications. If you have any questions, contact the medical affairs department of the manufacturer for the most recent prescribing information.

TO ENROLL

To enroll in the Sleep Medicines Clinic Continuing Medical Education program, call customer service at 1-800-654-2452 or sign up online at http://www.theclinics.com/home/cme. The CME program is available to subscribers for an additional annual fee of USD 126.

METHOD OF PARTICIPATION

In order to claim credit, participants must complete the following:

1. Complete enrolment as indicated above.
2. Read the activity.
3. Complete the CME Test and Evaluation. Participants must achieve a score of 70% on the test. All CME Tests and Evaluations must be completed online.

CME INQUIRIES/SPECIAL NEEDS

For all CME inquiries or special needs, please contact elsevierCME@elsevier.com.

Preface
FDG PET/CT: Normal Variations and Benign Findings - Translation to PET/MRI

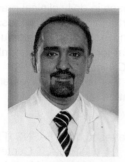

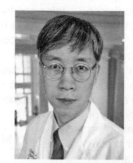

Mohsen Beheshti, MD, FASNC, FEBNM   Chun K. Kim, MD

Editors

F-18 fluorodeoxyglucose (FDG) is the most commonly used probe for PET imaging. Staging, restaging, and therapy monitoring are well-established clinical applications of the technique in various cancers. Variable retention of FDG is reported in different tumors based on their histopathologic differentiation and rate of glycolytic metabolism. FDG uptake also occurs in nonmalignant tissue, notably in the brain, thyroid gland, digestive tract, myocardium, skeletal muscle, bone marrow, and genitourinary tract. These sites of physiologic FDG activity are generally readily recognized; however, there are other common sites of variable physiologic and benign pathologic FDG uptake that could be confused with malignant neoplasms.

FDG is not a cancer-specific agent and its uptake is not uncommon in a number of inflammatory and infectious lesions, including sarcoidosis, tuberculosis, fungal infections, and cerebral abscesses. Furthermore, aging as well as different therapeutic procedures may affect the normal distribution of FDG and give place to different benign patterns of tracer uptake such as those observed in the healing bone, lymph nodes, joints, sites of infection, and aseptic inflammatory foci. Recognition and proper categorization of such physiologic variants and benign pathologic causes of FDG uptake are necessary for accurate interpretation of PET images.

To this end, many potential pitfalls and artefacts associated with FDG-PET imaging, which are very important to become familiar with to minimize false-positive diagnoses, have been reviewed in this issue of *PET Clinics*. Procedural standardization to include patient preparation, image acquisition, and processing as well as quantitative parameters utilized are necessary to minimize these potential pitfalls and artefacts so that accurate interpretation can be made.

Gamez-Cenzano and Pino-Sorroche provide an overview of the most important concepts related to standardization and quantification of FDG-PET images, focusing on the standardized uptake value and the potential errors that may arise when using this parameter in clinical practice. In addition, it provides useful recommendations to avoid or minimize errors with the standardization of imaging protocols.

Berti and coworkers expand on FDG-PET imaging of the brain. Intense tracer uptake is expected in the normal cerebral cortex and basal ganglia as glucose is the predominant substrate for brain metabolism. Accurate recognition of physiologic FDG distribution in the cortex, the effect of aging and of various treatments on cerebral FDG uptake, is of utmost importance when attempting to diagnose cognitive and tumoral brain disease.

In Hoejgaard and coworkers, Wachsmann and Gerbaudo, Zukotynski and Kim, Kohan and Avril

PET Clin 9 (2014) xiii–xiv

http://dx.doi.org/10.1016/j.cpet.2014.02.001

the authors expand on the multitude of causes responsible for FDG uptake in normal and benign pathologic findings in the head and neck, thorax, abdomen, and pelvis.

Grant concentrates on pediatric FDG-PET imaging. This specialized field of Nuclear Medicine imaging warrants additional skill and knowledge to be able to differentiate pediatric pathology and pathophysiology from benign processes particular to the pediatric population that may affect tracer distribution.

It is well known that the time interval between FDG injection and PET image acquisition affects the pattern and intensity of tracer uptake and its quantitation. In Cheng and coworkers, the authors shared their analysis of background activity rate of clearance from the various tissues by quantifying the FDG uptake at different times after tracer injection, to evaluate its clinical significance in each tissue type.

Radiotherapy may affect normal tissues and the pattern of FDG uptake within a radiation port, which may challenge the ability to differentiate postradiation changes from residual or recurrent tumor. To this end, Domachevsky and coworkers expand on postradiation (primarily external beam) histological and multimodality imaging findings with an emphasis on FDG-PET/CT.

Recently, hybrid PET and magnetic resonance imaging (MRI) have been introduced as a promising modality for whole body evaluation of oncology patients as well as for various other indications. Although current clinical experience is still in its infancy, Rakheja and coworkers review possible clinical indications of PET/MRI, especially in those situations in which PET/CT is of limited value.

In summary, this issue of *PET Clinics* provides important information to familiarize the reader with FDG patterns encountered in normal, benign pathologic conditions and in treatment-related sources of abnormal uptake, to minimize or avoid false-positive diagnoses in daily clinical practice.

We take this opportunity to thank Dr Abass Alavi for all his contributions in the field of molecular imaging and in particular for inviting us to contribute to this issue of *PET Clinics*.

We also dedicate this issue to our parents for their support, inspiration, and guidance.

Mohsen Beheshti, MD, FASNC, FEBNM
PET–CT Center LINZ
Department of Nuclear Medicine and
Endocrinology
St. Vincent's Hospital
Linz, Austria

Chun K. Kim, MD
Harvard Medical School
Division of Nuclear Medicine and
Molecular Imaging
Brigham and Women's Hospital
Boston, MA, USA

E-mail addresses:
Mohsen.Beheshti@bhs.at (M. Beheshti)
ckkim@bwh.harvard.edu (C.K. Kim)

Standardization and Quantification in FDG-PET/CT Imaging for Staging and Restaging of Malignant Disease

Cristina Gámez-Cenzano, MD, PhD[a],*,
Francisco Pino-Sorroche, PhD[b]

KEYWORDS

- PET/CT • FDG • Cancer • Quantification • Standardization • SUV • Quality control

KEY POINTS

- FDG-PET/CT is evolving from a valid qualitative clinical tool to a quantitative clinical and research tool.
- The requisites for quantification in FDG-PET/CT include standardization of protocols, equipment, QC procedures of the equipment, validated postprocessing software, and qualified staff.
- When using serial standardized uptake value measurements to assess response to therapy, imaging should be performed on the same scanner using the same image acquisition and reconstruction protocols.
- Various factors (technical, physical, and biological) affecting standardized uptake values should be taken into account in clinical practice to avoid misinterpretation of PET studies but it is crucial to control them in quantification.
- Participation in multicentric trials requires a qualification and following strictly predefined standardized protocols to reduce variability.

INTRODUCTION

[18]F-fluorodeoxyglucose (FDG) is a glucose analog that accumulates preferentially in malignant cells because of their higher glucose metabolism. PET/computed tomography with FDG (FDG-PET/CT) is routinely used for initial staging and follow-up in oncology patients with a proven value in most prevalent tumors, like lung cancer, breast cancer, colorectal cancer, and lymphoma. FDG uptake may help to distinguish malignant from benign lesions in some cases, except for some benign conditions such as inflammatory or infectious processes.[1] In general, higher-grade and less-differentiated tumors are associated with higher uptake of FDG as in lymphoma,[2] sarcoma,[3] and glioma.[4] In addition, higher accumulation is associated with poorer prognosis for some tumor types. Finally, response to treatment is correlated with a reduction or disappearance of FDG uptake in malignant lesions.[5]

Although visual interpretation of PET scans is the basis of the clinical report,[6] strategies to extract quantitative information will permit more objective diagnosis and comparisons between serial PET of a patient or among patient groups.

The authors have nothing to disclose.
[a] PET-Unit, Institut de Diagnòstic per la Imatge (IDI), Hospital Universitari de Bellvitge–IDIBELL, Av. Feixa Llarga, s/n, L'Hospitalet de Llobregat, Barcelona 08907, Spain; [b] Medical Physics Department, Institut Català d'Oncologia (ICO), Hospital Duran i Reynals–IDIBELL, Av Gran Via, 199-203, L'Hospitalet de Llobregat, Barcelona 08908, Spain
* Corresponding author.
E-mail address: cgamez@bellvitgehospital.cat

PET Clin 9 (2014) 117–127
http://dx.doi.org/10.1016/j.cpet.2013.10.003
1556-8598/14/$ – see front matter © 2014 Elsevier Inc. All rights reserved.

A major advantage of FDG-PET is the ability to quantify FDG accumulation in tissues and lesions. Absolute quantification usually requires long and complex dynamic PET acquisition protocols and accurate measurement of activity concentrations in arterial blood, which provides the input function to the kinetic model. Simplifications of these invasive techniques, involving normalization approaches or qualitative scales, have been applied with success.[5,7] Normalization approaches are based on the measured FDG concentration with regard to the injected FDG activity per weight obtaining a semiquantitative index. The most common parameter is called standardized uptake value (SUV) and it is described with more detail in a later section of this article.[5,7] In qualitative scales, lesion uptake is compared with the reference tissue uptake, usually the mediastinal blood pool or the liver, as in the assessment of early response to treatment in lymphoma (London or Deauville criteria).[8] The most used semiquantitative index in primary brain tumors is a lesion-to-reference ratio, using the normal white matter or the contralateral cortex as the reference tissue.[9]

Quantitative approaches have been proven to be successful in clinical routine practice, providing additional information of the aggressiveness of the primary tumor, helping the selection of the optimal site for biopsy in heterogeneous masses, as well as planning optimal field of radiotherapy. On the other hand, objective data of therapy efficacy are mandatory in clinical trials as final conclusions of such studies result in relevant regulatory and business decisions in drug development. Hence, quantitative assessment of therapy-induced changes is of great importance especially in multi-center clinical trials in which different institutions perform baseline PET/CT scans that should be compared with posttherapy scans.

This article reviews the most important concepts related to quantification with SUV measurements, how to assess response in oncology using SUV, the potential errors in SUV calculation and also provides useful recommendations to avoid or minimize errors with the standardization of protocols.

QUANTIFICATION WITH SUV MEASUREMENTS IN FDG-PET/CT STUDIES

SUV represents an index for FDG accumulation in tissue. Quantitative FDG-PET using SUV was introduced in the early 1990s by Strauss and Conti.[10] In 1993 Wahl and colleagues[11] published an initial report describing a rapid and significant decline in SUV in responder women with newly diagnosed breast cancer treated with chemo-

and/or hormonotherapy. Since then, numerous studies have been published showing the usefulness of SUV for monitoring response or predicting outcome in most FDG avid tumors.[12–15]

The SUV is a semiquantitative measure of normalized radioactivity concentration in PET images. To measure SUV, a 2D region of interest (ROI) or a 3D volume of interest (VOI) is positioned centrally within the tumor lesion using an interactive workstation. The measured radioactivity within the ROI/VOI is normalized to the average radioactivity in the body, which is approximated as the injected dose divided by the patient body weight (SUV_{bw}) or less frequently the patient lean body mass (SUV_{lbm} or SUL) or body surface area (SUV_{bsa}). The 2 common ways of reporting SUV are the mean or maximum of all voxels within the ROI known as SUV_{mean} and SUV_{max}, respectively. SUV_{mean} can be found also as SUV_{avrg}. Currently, SUV_{max} in a 3D VOI is the most recommended because it is less observer-dependent and more reproducible owing to the reason of independent ROI/VOI definition. SUV_{peak} is a hybrid measurement that includes a local average SUV value in a group of voxels surrounding the voxel with the highest activity; the concept is to maintain the reproducibility of SUV_{max} with improved statistics to reduce noise.[16] More recently, a different method of evaluating tumor metabolism has become readily available: total lesion glycolysis (TLG), which is an assessment of global metabolic activity in all viable cells throughout the lesion above a minimum threshold.[17] Unlike SUV_{max}, which reflects only the point of greatest metabolic activity within the tumor, it is hypothesized that TLG could better reflect tumor metabolic activity by taking into account the activity in the entire tumor (**Fig. 1**).[18]

ASSESSMENT OF TREATMENT RESPONSE IN ONCOLOGY WITH FDG-PET/CT USING SUV MEASUREMENTS

Current response evaluation criteria in solid tumors (RECIST) rely mainly on anatomic size of the tumor. The changes after treatment are categorized in 4 types of response: complete response, partial response, stable disease, and progressive disease.[19] The RECIST guidelines can be used successfully to monitor treatments that are able to shrink tumor lesions, such as cytotoxic agents. However, they have major limitations, especially in evaluating early effects to therapy or new targeted therapies where changes in size may not be visually evident. FDG-PET/CT allows an early assessment of treatment response and is a strong predictor of clinical outcome. Some

$$SUV_{bw} = \frac{activity\ concentration\ in\ tissue\ (mCi/ml)}{injected\ activity\ (mCi)/body\ weight\ (g)}\ in\ g/mL$$

$$SUV_{lbm} = SUL = \frac{activity\ concentration\ in\ tissue\ (mCi/ml)}{injected\ activity\ (mCi)/lean\_body\_mass(g)}\ in\ g/mL$$

$$SUV_{bsa} = \frac{activity\ concentration\ in\ tissue\ (mCi/ml)}{injected\ activity\ (mCi)/body\_surface\_area(cm^2)}\ in\ cm^2/mL$$

$$SUV_{mean} = SUV_{avrg} \qquad SUV_{max} \neq SUV_{peak}$$

$$TLG = SUVmean * Tumor\ Volume$$

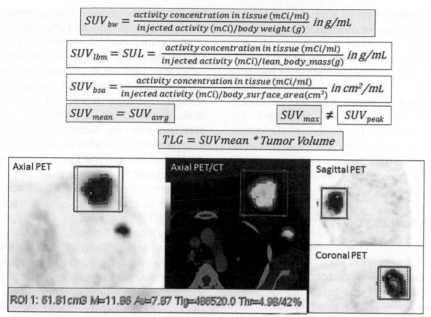

Fig. 1. SUV measurements. The FDG-PET/CT images show a VOI centered on a breast tumor. Volume (in cm^3), SUV$_{max}$ (M), SUV$_{mean}$ (Av), TLG (Tlg), and Threshold (Thr) have been calculated using an Advantage workstation (GE Healthcare). The blue mark within the tumor indicates the voxel with the highest activity.

relevant examples are aggressive lymphoma (interim PET for early evaluation during chemotherapy)[20,21] and gastrointestinal tract sarcomas treated with imatinib[22] but it also occurs in many other tumors.[18] Quantitative PET plays an important role in this scenario and it is being considered as a "qualified biomarker."[23] Metabolic response in solid tumors has been defined using SUV according to the European Organization for Research and Treatment of Cancer (EORTC) criteria[5] and more recently the PET Response Criteria in Solid Tumors (PERCIST) criteria.[24] A simplified comparative summary is presented in **Table 1.**

Table 1
Imaging assessment of response in oncology

Response Criteria	RECIST 1.1	EORTC	PERCIST 1.0
Main parameters	Sum of longest diameters of measurable lesions (5/total and 2/organ)	SUV$_{bw}$	SUL (>liver), TLG 5 more active measurable lesions (2/organ)
CR (CMR)	Disappearance of all previous lesions	Disappearance of all previous active lesions	Disappearance of all previous active lesions
PR (PMR)	Tumors shrink >30%	↓SUV ≥15% (1st cycle) or 25% (≥2 cycles) No ↑extent of tumor	↓SUL ≥30% (≥0.8 units) No ↑ extent of tumor
PD (PMD)	Tumors grow >20% New lesions	↑SUV ≥25% ↑extent of tumor >20% New lesions	↑SUL ≥30% (≥0.8 units) ↑extent of tumor (TLG >75%) New lesions
SD (SMD)	Between PR and PD	Between PMR and PMD	Between PMR and PMD

Abbreviations: CMR, complete metabolic response; CR, complete response; PD, progressive disease; PMD, progressive metabolic disease; PMR, partial metabolic response; PR, partial response; SD, stable disease; SMD, stable metabolic disease; SUL, SUV normalized to the lean body mass.

The development of more individualized thera-pies, such as the use of molecular-based drugs, requires specific protocols to improve detection and to assess the effects of the treatment as early as possible. Due to ineffective therapies that may allow a change in the treatment and outcome of patients, the use of these so-called response-adaptative or risk-adaptative treatment ap-proaches is expected to increase.[25] Therefore, reliable SUV measurements are essential when evaluating response to therapy and it is critically important to guarantee the most accurate and comparable values.

QUANTIFICATION IN FDG-PET: THE REQUISITES

The requisites for quantification in FDG-PET/CT include standardization of protocols, quality con-trol (QC) procedures of equipment, image quality analysis, adequate postprocessing tools, and qualified staff.

Standardization

Standardization of protocols is crucial to guar-antee reproducibility and to minimize errors. Reproducibility is an essential factor to compare studies for the same patient–same hospital or be-tween different institutions. Some relevant guide-lines have been published. One of the most recent reviews that integrates the previous ones corresponds to the European Association of Nu-clear Medicine procedure guidelines.[26]

QC Procedures

QC procedures mainly verify the correct acquisi-tion and reconstruction of PET/CT images. They must be performed on a regular basis and after every significant maintenance of the equipment. Furthermore, they should be included within a quality management system with registration of all performed tests, calibrations, and preventive and corrective actions.

It is essential to perform dose calibrator test pro-cedures correctly because image quality, accurate quantification, and patient safety highly depend on the reliability of this instrument. The required tests are accuracy, constancy, linearity, and geometry. The constancy test, performed at installation and thereafter daily, measures instrument precision and is designed to show that reproducible read-ings are obtained the day after using a long-lived source (eg,[137]Cs). The linearity test, performed at installation and quarterly, is designed to prove that the dose calibrator readout is linear for sour-ces varying from the microcurie range through to the megacurie range. The geometry test, per-formed at installation and after repair, is designed to show that correct readings can be obtained regardless of the sample size or geometry. Accu-racy tests, performed at installation and annually, are designed to show that the calibrator is giving correct readings throughout the entire energy scale likely to be encountered using different standard sources. Based on Nuclear Regulatory Commission requirements, a maximum of ±10% deviation between standard and expected values is acceptable for all dose calibrator tests.[27]

QC procedures of the PET/CT scanner make it possible to check (and even correct after some tests) PET image quality, CT image quality and patient dose, CT-based attenuation correction accuracy, and CT and PET co-registration accu-racy. They can be found in published standard descriptions[28] and national and international pro-tocols.[29–31] All manufacturers supply test proce-dures; phantoms test and specific software should also be taken into account when writing local operating procedures. In the specific case of the CT scanner, as a radiograph device, it must also be checked according to national radia-tion safety legislation. The most important tests include the CT daily QC, the PET daily QC, PET normalization, and cross-calibration (well counter). The PET daily QC test checks detectors normally using a [68]Ge source or phantom. In PET normaliza-tion the [68]Ge source or phantom is used to acquire crystal efficiency data for correcting detector non-uniformities and is applied to the following acquisi-tions. The aim of the cross-calibration test of the PET/CT scanner is to determine the correct cali-bration of the scanner with the institution's own dose calibrator and should be performed quar-terly. It uses the PET/CT image data of a fillable phantom with water whereby a recommended ac-tivity of FDG has been injected according to the manufacturer's specifications. This calibration is applied in reconstruction of clinical PET studies to obtain SUV measurements. An optional test[29] the authors are performing in their institution is an additional acquisition of the phantom when calculated FDG activity is approximately 1 mCi using the clinical protocol of the system for the acquisition and reconstruction of a 2-bed whole-body study (entering also the weight of the phan-tom). In the analysis of images, SUV in the center of the phantom should be 1 ± 0.1. This test is frequently requested to be sent to central labora-tories to be qualified in multicentric clinical trials (Fig. 2). Although image reconstruction algorithms depend on the manufacturer scanner, they should be chosen so that they meet specifications for both calibration QC and image quality/SUV

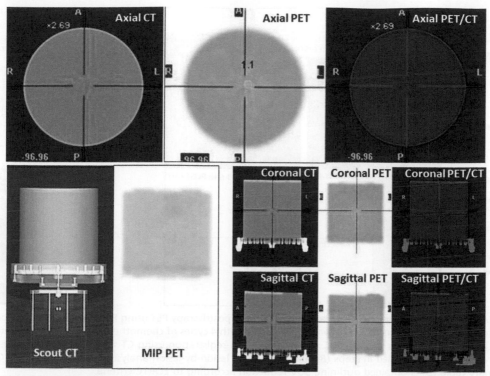

Fig. 2. Phantom acquisition to check SUV. Images of a PET/CT acquisition of a plastic cylinder filled with water and 1 mCi of FDG are shown. SUV_{max} in the center is 1.1 within the accepted range 1 ± 0.1. MIP, maximum intensity projection.

recovery QC.[26] In addition, a preventive maintenance must be performed by the manufacturer every 3 to 6 months.

Other additional minor equipment must also be monitored. *All clocks*, including the one in the PET/CT system, should be synchronized with the official local time within 1 minute and checked frequently. *Weighing scales* should be accredited and checked at least annually. *Glucometers* are used to check the blood glucose level before FDG administration. Presently there are 2 approaches for carrying out glucometer QC. The first is based on the comparison of results obtained by a controlled glucose meter and the use of the laboratory method or point-of-care testing device as a surrogate reference analyzer. The second one is a traditionally organized external quality assessment scheme with the use of a dedicated control material. The recommended permissible measurement error can be realistically set at 10%.[32] In their institution the authors use the second approach quarterly for every glucometer. Not a glucometer or a similar bedside device, but a blood glucose test must be performed with a calibrated and validated method if plasma glucose level is used as correction of SUV measurements.[33]

Multilesion approach in serial PET studies is optimized using *validated semiautomated image-based PET/CT analysis programs* now produced by various manufacturers.[34] Such programs enable physicians to assess changes in tumor activity and size across several time points, as part of therapy response evaluation by comparing quantitative values of diameters and SUV measurements for morphologic/CT criteria (RECIST and World Health Organization) and metabolic/PET criteria (EORTC and PERCIST). These solutions present the additional advantages of being a more accurate and reproducible intra- and interobserver than one-by-one study analysis. PET volume computer-assisted reading, an application of the Advantage Workstation (General Electric Healthcare, Milwaukee, WI, EEUU), is one such program that is used in the authors' institution and incorporates precise examination-to-examination coregistration, using the companion CT scan as a fiduciary marker, and threshold-based image segmentation (**Fig. 3**).

Qualification of Personnel

The team of professionals should include qualified physicians, technologists, and medical physicists.

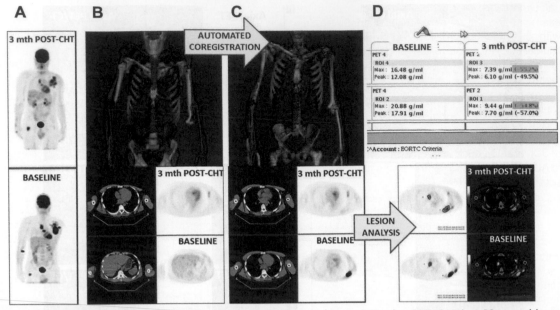

Fig. 3. A comparative analysis between a baseline PET and posttherapy PET using PETVCAR in a 38-year-old man with undifferentiated cancer of unknown origin treated with 4 cycles of chemotherapy (CDDP and pemetrexed). MIP PET images are shown in column *A*. An automated co-registration using CT structures in the 2 time points (*green and red*) is performed in steps (*B*) to (*C*). Finally, a lesion-by-lesion analysis is performed with VOIs and a summary table (*D*) is obtained outlining SUV reduction according to EORTC criteria.

Quality management system should include proper training of all the staff involved in the correct and safe use of the equipment and its QC procedures and a clear definition of responsibilities. This aspect has been reviewed in several guidelines.[29,31]

ERRORS IN QUANTIFICATION IN FDG-PET/CT: WHAT CAN WE DO?

Factors affecting quantification (SUVs) and their impact have been discussed extensively in numerous articles. Briefly, errors have been categorized as technical, physical, and biological (**Fig. 4**),[16,35] which are explained in the following section to avoid or minimize their impact.

Technical Errors: What Can We Do?

Errors relating to FDG administration procedure constitute up to 50% of technical errors, with a high impact on SUV calculation, most times with no or difficult solutions.[35] In paravenous injection (extravasation) the net FDG administered dose is reduced, resulting in incorrect underestimated SUV. Due to omitting the injection site from the acquisition, FDG extravasation is underreported. Extravasation should not only be avoided but also reported to explain that SUV cannot be

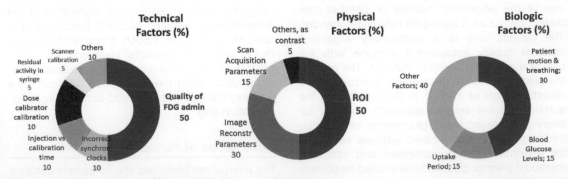

Fig. 4. Overview of factors affecting FDG-PET quantification.

calculated and to avoid false interpretations of the examination.[36–38] In some clinical trials, studies with extravasation may be excluded. Complex clinical trials even request an additional acquisition of injection site to check this aspect to apply automated methods for dose correction[39] but this approach has not been implemented in routine clinical practice.[40]

Regarding FDG activity, recommendations are based on the system, the protocol acquisition (2D or 3D), and the patient weight. In general, adhering to ALARA principles, it is preferable to use reduced activity increasing scan duration. Some clinical trials indicate the FDG dose to be administered in every scan. In the authors' institution, a dose of 0.1 mCi (3.7 MBq)/kg of weight is generally administered in routine and multicenter studies. It is a practical solution within all recommended ranges and it is very easy for technologists to bear in mind: a patient of 80 kg needs a dose of 8 mCi; a patient of 65 kg needs 6.5 mCi, and so on.

In the case of manual administration of FDG, a triple-channel system is highly recommended for administering it and afterward flushing with at least 10 mL of physiologic saline (NaCl 0.9%). In the case of automated administration, the user must verify that the automated system and procedures assure a real administered FDG activity within 3% accuracy. Residual activity in syringe (or administration system) must be measured to use exact administered dose for SUV calculations. A lower net dose results in incorrect lower SUV. This error represents approximately 5%.

The recommended interval between FDG administration and the start of acquisition is 60 minutes. However, for certain clinical trials this may change depending on the disease and aims of the study. FDG dose at the time of preparation (calibration), time of injection, and the start of acquisition must be recorded carefully with synchronized clocks. Incorrect synchronization of clocks of the dose calibrator and PET/CT scanner has been reported by 10%. A wrong time interval between injection versus calibration results in incorrect SUV because that interval is used for decay correction of administered dose and can affect the SUV value in up to 10% of cases.

When repeating a scan on the same patient, especially in the context of therapy response assessment, it is essential to inject the same FDG dose (tolerance ± 10%) and to apply the same interval between injection time and the beginning of acquisition (tolerance ± 5 minutes).

Error in relative calibration between PET scanner and dose calibration represents 10% but can be easily controlled by the cross-calibration test previously described.

Physical Errors: What Can We Do?

Physical errors are mostly determined by the acquisition parameters (up to 15%), reconstruction parameters (up to 30%), and the ROI (up to 55%).

CT and PET acquisition and reconstruction parameters must be the ones provided and recommended by the manufacturer. The CT data that are acquired during the PET/CT scanning session are usually reconstructed by use of filtered back projection or a similar algorithm. The PET emission data must be corrected for geometric response and detector efficiency (normalization), system dead time, random coincidences, scatter, and attenuation. Some of these corrections (for example, attenuation correction) can be directly applied in the reconstruction process. In serial scans of the same patient the same PET/CT system and identical acquisition and reconstruction settings must be applied.

SUV outcome strongly depends on size and type of used ROI/VOI defined in a software program. An ROI/VOI should be defined for every lesion in axial plane on original reconstructed PET images with attenuation correction centered on the tumor area with highest uptake. In clinical environments such programs are considered medical devices and validated and US -Food and Drug Administration or European Union Centers of Excellence certified versions are needed. In recent years, there has been a huge amount of image analysis software made freely available to the public. Free software is advantageous by providing open accessibility and research in imaging analysis tools. However, it is the user's responsibility to verify that the software is well documented, validated, and kept up-to-date to ensure that the quality requirements of the particular task are met.[41] Some free software services provide a certified version available commercially, usually with extra cost. Additional errors are found when 2D ROIs that are not drawn on multiple axial slices covering the whole lesion to determine the highest activity. Therefore, 3D VOI is preferable but not only axial, but also coronal and sagittal planes should be checked to avoid including adjacent FDG avid structures (bladder, heart). Lesions smaller than 10 mm should not be quantified due to inaccuracy attributable to the "clinical" scanner resolution, so-called partial-volume effect causing underestimation of the SUV measurements.[16,42,43] Because different software platforms or programs provide different SUV outcomes, even when identical data sets are used, standardization of ROI methodology and data analysis software is urgently needed. At present, some initiatives, such as that of the Quantitative Imaging Biomarkers Alliance, are being undertaken to address these issues. Alternatively, in the absence of standardized ROI software and implementation, quantification of FDG PET studies in a multicenter setting may need to be reviewed and analyzed centrally.[35]

The remaining physical errors (5%) are related to the use of contrast agents during CT for PET Attenuation Correction and the use of different SUV corrections. High-density contrast agents may produce an overestimation of attenuation and therefore higher uptake (higher SUV) may occur but the recommendations are controversial. Some authors support the use of contrast-enhanced CT for PET attenuation correction.[44,45] Protocol acquisition of FDG-PET/CT of clinical trials specifies the permission or prohibition of IV contrast injection in the CT portion for attenuation correction.

Unusual errors are found when comparing different SUV measurements (for example, SUV_{max} to SUV_{mean}, SUV_{bw} to SUV_{lbm}, or mixing SUV_{max} with SUV_{peak}). SUV blood glucose level correction is very risky. High blood glucose levels cause underestimation of SUV; the use of serum glucose level correction in SUV equation results in different SUV outcomes that are only valid if a blood validated test, but not a glucometer, has been used to check the blood glucose level before FDG injection. If blood glucose levels are high (usually >120 mg/dL), most guidelines do not recommend SUV correction; other recommended approaches are to reschedule the PET study or insulin administration.[26]

Biological Errors: What Can We Do?

Biological factors include errors mainly due to patient motion and breathing (30%), patient high glucose level (15%), and too long or different uptake periods (15%).

Patient motion and breathing cause many image artifacts as a result of mismatches in positions between CT-AC and PET emission scans. Lower SUV may result from respiratory motion (resolution loss) especially in lung bases and upper abdomen. Unwanted patient motion can be minimized by improving patient comfort (immobilization devices) and patient information (clear instructions not to move, to breathe shallowly).[46] Respiratory motion correction approaches include specific acquisition protocols (breath-holding in quiet-end-expiration)[46] and hardware and software solutions.[47]

High blood glucose level with FDG injection can seriously reduce SUV measurement because of the reduction of FDG cell uptake in its competition with glucose.[16] Some specific recommendations

apply to patients with diabetes mellitus so as to achieve normal glycemic values before the PET study.[26] Depending on patient circumstances and the trial being conducted, the PET study can be rescheduled, the patient can be excluded from that trial, or the administration of insulin can be considered.[26]

As previously described, most guidelines recommend an uptake period of 60 ± 10 minutes.[26] Higher SUVs occur at increasing time intervals between injection and start of the PET acquisition; this has been used in some clinical settings to increase the lesion uptake when surrounding normal tissue shows a high uptake of FDG (as in the brain or liver) and in dual-time protocols.[48,49]

Other biological errors (40%) can be related to patients' weight, peritumoral inflammation, and individual therapy-induced changes. If SUV is used in monitoring response, then weight should be measured with the same calibrated scale at the PET facility, not on self-reported weight or from the patient chart.[16]

FDG-PET/CT IN MULTICENTRIC CLINICAL TRIALS

Standardization of protocols in PET/CT centers facilitates participation in multicentric clinical trials.

There are several kinds of PET/CT accreditation bodies that grant acceptance of PET/CT centers after a technical evaluation of the site information: equipment (including quality assurance [QA]), capabilities of electronic transfer, and the standard of care. The submission of a phantom scan is usually required periodically to check accuracy of the scanner SUV calibration.[50,51]

Official accreditation by scientific societies in the United States[51] and the European Union[52,53] is highly recommended but is not a requisite because most clinical trials collaborate with a central laboratory in charge of qualifying PET centers and central image analysis.

SUMMARY AND NEXT STEPS

FDG-PET/CT is evolving from a valid qualitative clinical tool to a quantitative clinical and research tool.

The present article reviews the requisites for quantification in FDG-PET/CT that include standardization of protocols, equipment QC procedures of the equipment, validated postprocessing software, and qualified staff. When using serial SUV measurements to assess response to therapy, imaging should be performed on the same scanner using the same image acquisition and reconstruction protocols. Various factors (technical, physical, and biological) affecting SUVs have been described. These factors should be taken into account in clinical practice to avoid misinterpretation of PET studies but it is crucial to control them in quantification. Participation in multicentric trials requires a qualification and following strictly predefined standardized protocols to reduce variability.

The main challenges in the near future will be to improve reproducibility (between scanners, analysis workstations, PET centers) and to implement quantitative metabolic response criteria in routine therapeutic decision-making.

ACKNOWLEDGMENTS

We would like to thank all the professionals involved in standardization and quantification in our institution. We are very grateful to Manel Roca, M. Angels Hernández, and Rafael Puchal for their contribution in setting up and maintaining the standardized protocols in radiopharmacy. We would also like to thank Cristina Picón and Ismael Sancho from the Medical Physics Department for their support. Finally, we would like to express much appreciation for the commitment of physicians, technologists, and administrative personnel of the PET unit to achieve quality accreditation (ISO 9001) and make reliable quantification possible for routine and research PET studies.

REFERENCES

1. Fletcher JW, Djulbegovic B, Soares HP, et al. Recommendations on the use of 18F-FDG PET in oncology. J Nucl Med 2008;49(3):480–508.
2. Schöder H, Noy A, Gönen M, et al. Intensity of 18fluorodeoxyglucose uptake in positron emission tomography distinguishes between indolent and aggressive non-Hodgkin's lymphoma. J Clin Oncol 2005;23(21):4643–51.
3. Rakheja R, Makis W, Skamene S, et al. Correlating metabolic activity on 18F-FDG PET/CT with histopathologic characteristics of osseous and soft-tissue sarcomas: a retrospective review of 136 patients. AJR Am J Roentgenol 2012;198(6):1409–16.
4. Kosaka N, Tsuchida T, Uematsu H, et al. 18F-FDG PET of common enhancing malignant brain tumors. AJR Am J Roentgenol 2008;190(6):W365–9.
5. Young H, Baum R, Cremerius U, et al. Measurement of clinical and subclinical tumour response using [18F]-fluorodeoxyglucose and positron emission tomography: review and 1999 EORTC recommendations. European organization for research and treatment of cancer (EORTC) PET study group. Eur J Cancer 1999;35:1773–82.
6. Coleman RE. Is quantitation necessary for oncological PET studies? For. Eur J Nucl Med Mol Imaging 2002;29(1):133–5.
7. Vriens D, Visser EP, de Geus-Oei LF, et al. Methodological considerations in quantification of oncological FDG PET studies. Eur J Nucl Med Mol Imaging 2010;37(7):1408–25.
8. Meignan M, Gallamini A, Haioun C. Report on the first international workshop on interim-PET scan in lymphoma. Leuk Lymphoma 2009;50:1257–60.
9. Tripathi M, Sharma R, Varshney R, et al. Comparison of F-18 FDG and C-11 methionine PET/CT for the evaluation of recurrent primary brain tumors. Clin Nucl Med 2012;37(2):158–63.
10. Strauss LG, Conti PS. The applications of PET in clinical oncology. J Nucl Med 1991;32(4):623–48 [discussion: 649–50].
11. Wahl RL, Zasadny K, Helvie M, et al. Metabolic monitoring of breast cancer chemohormonotherapy using positron emission tomography: initial evaluation. J Clin Oncol 1993;11(11):2101–11.
12. Tateishi U, Gamez C, Dawood S, et al. Bone metastases in patients with metastatic breast cancer: morphologic and metabolic monitoring of response to systemic therapy with integrated PET/CT. Radiology 2008;247(1):189–96.
13. Okereke IC, Gangadharan SP, Kent MS, et al. Standard uptake value predicts survival in non-small cell lung cancer. Ann Thorac Surg 2009;88(3):911–5 [discussion: 915–6].
14. Namura K, Minamimoto R, Yao M, et al. Impact of maximum standardized uptake value (SUVmax) evaluated by 18-Fluoro-2-deoxy-D-glucose positron emission tomography/computed tomography (18F-FDG-PET/CT) on survival for patients with advanced renal cell carcinoma: a preliminary report. BMC Cancer 2010;10:667.
15. Miyazaki Y, Nawa Y, Miyagawa M, et al. Maximum standard uptake value of 18F-fluorodeoxyglucose positron emission tomography is a prognostic factor for progression-free survival of newly diagnosed patients with diffuse large B cell lymphoma. Ann Hematol 2013;92(2):239–44.
16. Adams MC, Turkington TG, Wilson JM, et al. A systematic review of the factors affecting accuracy of SUV measurements. AJR Am J Roentgenol 2010;195(2):310–20.
17. Larson SM, Erdi Y, Akhurst T, et al. Tumor treatment response based on visual and quantitative changes in global tumor glycolysis using PET-FDG imaging. The visual response score and the change in total lesion glycolysis. Clin Positron Imaging 1999;2(3):159–71.
18. Costelloe CM, Macapinlac HA, Madewell JE, et al. 18F-FDG PET/CT as an indicator of

progression-free and overall survival in osteosarcoma. J Nucl Med 2009;50(3):340–7.

19. Eisenhauer EA, Therasse P, Bogaerts J, et al. New response evaluation criteria in solid tumours: revised RECIST guideline (version 1.1). Eur J Cancer 2009;45(2):228–47.

20. Moskowitz CH. Interim PET-CT in the management of diffuse large B-cell lymphoma. Hematology Am Soc Hematol Educ Program 2012;2012:397–401.

21. Cortés Romera M, Gámez Cenzano C, Caresia Aróztegui AP, et al. Utilidad de la PET-TC en la valoración de la respuesta precoz al tratamiento en el linfoma B difuso de célula grandes. Resultados preliminares. Rev Esp Med Nucl Imagen Mol 2012;31(3):135–41 [in Spanish].

22. Treglia G, Mirk P, Stefanelli A, et al. 18F-fluorodeoxyglucose positron emission tomography in evaluating treatment response to imatinib or other drugs in gastrointestinal stromal tumors: a systematic review. Clin Imaging 2012;36(3):167–75.

23. Larson SM, Schwartz LH. 18F-FDG PET as a candidate for "qualified biomarker": functional assessment of treatment response in oncology. J Nucl Med 2006;47(6):901–3.

24. Wahl RL, Jacene H, Kasamon Y, et al. From RECIST to PERCIST: evolving considerations for PET response criteria in solid tumours. J Nucl Med 2009;50(Suppl 1):122S–50S.

25. Moskowitz CH, Schöder H, Teruya-Feldstein J, et al. Risk-adapted dose-dense immunochemotherapy determined by interim FDG-PET in advanced-stage diffuse large B-Cell lymphoma. J Clin Oncol 2010;28:1896–903.

26. Boellaard R, O'Doherty MJ, Weber WA, et al. FDG PET and PET/CT: EANM procedure guidelines for tumour PET imaging: version 1.0. Eur J Nucl Med Mol Imaging 2010;37(1):181–200.

27. The American Association of Physicist in Medicine. The selection, use, calibration, and quality assurance of radionuclide calibrators used in nuclear medicine. REPORT NO. 181. College Park, MD: AAPM; 2012.

28. National Electrical Manufacturers Association. National Electrical Manufacturers Association. NEMA Standards Publication NU 2-1994. Performance measurements of positron emission tomographs. Washington, DC: National Electrical Manufacturers Association; 1994. p. 2001–7.

29. International Atomic Energy Agency. Quality assurance for PET and PET/CT Systems IAEA Human Health Series No. 1, Vienna: International Atomic Energy Agency. 2009.

30. EANM Physics Committee, Busemann Sokole E, Płachcínska A, Britten A, et al. Routine quality control recommendations for nuclear medicine instrumentation. Eur J Nucl Med Mol Imaging 2010; 37(3):662–71.

31. Delbeke D, Coleman RE, Guiberteau MJ, et al. Procedure guideline for tumor imaging with 18F-FDG PET/CT 1.0. J Nucl Med 2006;47(5):885–95.

32. Solnica B, Naskalsk JW. Quality control of self-monitoring of blood glucose: why and how? J Diabetes Sci Technol 2007;1(2):164–8.

33. Dai KS, Tai DY, Ho P, et al. Accuracy of the Easytouch blood glucose self-monitoring system: a study of 516 cases. Clin Chim Acta 2004;349: 135–41.

34. Fox JJ, Autran-Blanc E, Morris MJ, et al. Practical approach for comparative analysis of multilesion molecular imaging using a semiautomated program for PET/CT. J Nucl Med 2011;52(11):1727–32.

35. Boellaard R. Standards for PET image acquisition and quantitative data analysis. J Nucl Med 2009; 50(Suppl 1):11S–20S.

36. Osman MM, Muzaffar R, Altinyay ME, et al. FDG dose extravasations in PET/CT: frequency and impact on SUV measurements. Front Oncol 2011; 1(41):1–6.

37. Manohar K, Agrawal K, Bhattacharya A, et al. New axillary lymph nodal F-18 fluoro-deoxy glucose uptake in an interim positron emission tomography scan – not always a sign of disease progression. Indian J Nucl Med 2011;26(4): 192–3.

38. Sonoda LI, Ghosh-Ray S, Sanghera B, et al. FDG injection site extravasation: potential pitfall of misinterpretation and missing metastases. Clin Nucl Med 2012;37(11):1115–6.

39. Miyashita K, Takahashi N, Oka T, et al. SUV correction for injection errors in FDG-PET examination. Ann Nucl Med 2007;21(10):607–13.

40. Hall N, Zhang J, Reid R, et al. Impact of FDG extravasation on SUV measurements in clinical PET/CT. Should we routinely scan the injection site? J Nucl Med 2006;47(Suppl 1):115P (meeting abstract).

41. de la Prieta R. Free software for pet imaging, positron emission tomography - current clinical and research aspects. In: Hsieh CH, editor. 2012. ISBN: 978-953-307-824-3, InTech, doi:10.5772/31882. Available at: http://www.intechopen.com/books/positron-emission-tomography-current-clinical-and-research-aspects/free-software-for-pet-imaging. Accessed 2012.

42. Soret M, Bacharach SL, Buvat I. Partial-volume effect in PET tumor imaging. J Nucl Med 2007; 48(6):932–45.

43. Shankar LK, Hoffman JM, Bacharach S, et al. Consensus recommendations for the use of 18F-FDG PET as an indicator of therapeutic response in patients in National Cancer Institute Trials. J Nucl Med 2006;47(6):1059–66.

44. Berthelsen AK, Holm S, Loft A, et al. PET/CT with intravenous contrast can be used for PET

attenuation correction in cancer patients. Eur J Nucl Med Mol Imaging 2005;32:1167–75.

45. Yau YY, Chan WS, Tam YM, et al. Application of intravenous contrast in PET/CT: does it really introduce significant attenuation correction error? J Nucl Med 2005;46:283–91.

46. Wong TZ, Paulson EK, Nelson RC, et al. Practical approach to diagnostic CT combined with PET. AJR Am J Roentgenol 2007;188(3):622–9.

47. Rahmim A, Rousset O, Zaidi H. Strategies for motion tracking and correction in PET. PET Clin 2007;2(2):251–66.

48. Lee JW, Kim SK, Lee SM, et al. Detection of hepatic metastases using dual-time-point FDG PET/CT scans in patients with colorectal cancer. Mol Imaging Biol 2011;13(3):565–72.

49. Schillaci O. Use of dual-point fluorodeoxyglucose imaging to enhance sensitivity and specificity. Semin Nucl Med 2012;42(4):267–80.

50. Westerterp M, Pruim J, Oyen W, et al. Quantification of FDG PET studies using standardised uptake values in multi-centre trials: effects of image reconstruction, resolution and ROI definition parameters. Eur J Nucl Med Mol Imaging 2007; 34(3):392–404.

51. Scheuermann JS, Saffer JR, Karp JS, et al. Qualification of PET scanners for use in multicenter cancer clinical trials: the American College of Radiology Imaging Network experience. J Nucl Med 2009;50(7):1187–93.

52. Boellaard R, Oyen WJ, Hoekstra CJ, et al. The Netherlands protocol for standardisation and quantification of FDG whole body PET studies in multi-centre trials. Eur J Nucl Med Mol Imaging 2008;35:2320–33.

53. Boellaard R, Hristova I, Ettinger S, et al. Initial experience with the EANM accreditation procedure of FDG PET/CT devices. Eur J Cancer 2011; 47(Suppl 4):S8 (meeting abstract).

Brain
Normal Variations and Benign Findings in Fluorodeoxyglucose-PET/Computed Tomography Imaging

Valentina Berti, MD, PhD[a],*, Lisa Mosconi, PhD[b], Alberto Pupi, MD[a]

KEYWORDS

- 18F-FDG-PET • Normal brain • Normal variants • Aging brain • Medications effect • Artifacts

KEY POINTS

- Brain 18F-fluorodeoxyglucose (18F-FDG) PET allows the in vivo study of cerebral glucose metabolism, reflecting neuronal and synaptic activity.
- 18F-FDG-PET has been extensively used to detect metabolic alterations in several neurologic diseases compared with normal aging; however, healthy subjects have variants of 18F-FDG distribution, especially as associated with aging.
- Healthy aging is associated with mild cortical hypometabolism involving preferentially the frontal lobes; in particular anterior cingulate cortex, dorsolateral and medial prefrontal cortices, and orbitofrontal cortex.
- 18F-FDG uptake in the normal brain could be affected by several substances and medications, including caffeine, alcohol, abused drugs such as amphetamines and cocaine, sedatives, neuroleptics, corticosteroids, and chemotherapy agents.
- Several artifacts may influence 18F-FDG brain distribution and cause interpretation errors.

INTRODUCTION

Glucose is the main metabolic substrate of the brain and its oxidation produces the amount of energy that is necessary for adequate cerebral activity.

The PET tracer 18F-fluorodeoxyglucose (18F-FDG) allows the in vivo study of glucose metabolism, and since its introduction in 1976 it has been the most widely used PET tracer in both clinical and research settings.[1]

The local glucose consumption, and thus 18F-FDG cerebral uptake, correlates strictly with local neuronal activity, and proportionally increases with stimulus intensity or frequency[2] or decreases in conditions of sensory deprivation.[3] Such metabolic variations take place at the level of synaptic connections.[4] As such, neurotransmission and signal transduction are the processes with the highest energy requirements. It has been estimated that the energy demand of neurotransmission and related events exceeds 80% of total cerebral energy consumption.[5]

Connections between neurons are performed mainly by excitatory glutamatergic synapses, which

This work was supported in part by National Institute of Health/National Institute on Aging 5R01AG035137 and Alzheimer's Association IIRG-09-132030 (L. Mosconi).

a Nuclear Medicine Unit, Department of Biomedical, Experimental and Clinical Sciences, University of Florence, Largo Brambilla, 3, Florence 50134, Italy; b Center for Brain Health, New York University School of Medicine, 145 East 32nd Street, 5th Floor, Room 5122, New York, NY 10016, USA
* Corresponding author.
E-mail address: valentina.berti@unifi.it

account for most all the cortical synapses, yielding an energy consumption of around 80% of total cortical consumption.[5]

A large body of literature shows that 18F-FDG-PET adds value to diagnostic evaluation of several neurologic diseases. In particular, 18F-FDG-PET substantially improves diagnostic accuracy and differential diagnosis, and enables earlier and better treatment planning of neurodegenerative disorders.[6,7]

Although most studies have focused on detection of abnormal, disease-specific 18F-FDG distribution patterns, little is known about brain glucose metabolism in clinically and cognitively normal, healthy individuals, and about normal variants of 18F-FDG uptake in this population.

Thorough knowledge of the normal variants of brain function, occurring in healthy aging or related to gender, is critical for detection of abnormal findings and for investigating neurologic diseases.

This article focuses on 18F-FDG-PET findings in so-called normal brain aging, and in particular on metabolic differences occurring with aging and as a function of gender. The effects of different substances, medications, and therapy procedures are discussed, as well as common artifacts.

IMAGING TECHNIQUE

Updated procedure guidelines for 18F-FDG-PET brain imaging were published by the Society of Nuclear Medicine in 2009[8] and include all relevant information to be collected during the procedure, instructions for patient's management and preparation for PET scanning, and a summary of the standardized acquisition protocol. These topics are summarized in **Boxes 1–3**, respectively.

18F-FDG-PET images should be reconstructed in transaxial, coronal, and sagittal planes.

Box 2
Patient preparation before PET scanning

Fasting for at least 4 to 6 hours

Oral hydration with water should be encouraged

Avoid caffeine, alcohol, or drugs that may affect cerebral glucose metabolism

Check blood glucose level (ideally not greater than 150–200 mg/dL)

Environmental conditions: resting state, patient with eyes open and ears unoccluded in a quiet, dimly lit room, with minimal background noise

Start intravenous line for 18F-FDG administration (at least 10 minutes before tracer injection)

For a comprehensive evaluation of brain 18F-FDG-PET images, all 3 projection planes should be used. The transaxial plane is recommended for evaluation of all cortical and subcortical structures. Transaxial images should be reoriented both along the anterior commissure–posterior commissure (AC-PC) line and temporal long axis (for better assessment of the temporal lobe) (**Fig. 1**). The coronal plane is recommended for inspection of posterior cingulate, angular gyri, and medial temporal lobes (including hippocampal areas). The sagittal plane is valuable in evaluations of the frontal and temporal poles.

NORMAL ANATOMY

Glucose is the only source of energy of the brain, which is known to account for as much as 20% of total-body glucose metabolism in the fasting

---

Box 1
Relevant patient history and data

Focused history: head trauma, known neurologic or psychiatric disorders, brain tumors, prior brain operations

Clinical history: patient complaints, neurologic/psychiatric examination, mental status examination (Mini-Mental State Examination, neuropsychological tests), cognitive impairment

Recent morphologic imaging studies (eg, computed tomography, magnetic resonance imaging, or prior PET or single-photon computed tomography brain studies)

Current medications

Box 3
Acquisition protocol

Administered dose	185–370 MBq
Acquisition starting time	30 minutes after injection 60 minutes after injection (oncology)
During acquisition	Well-tolerated head immobilization procedures should be implemented, to minimize head movements
Acquisition duration	20 minutes (depending on PET equipment and patient compliance)
Reconstruction	Transaxial matrix size: 128 × 128 or 256 × 256 Typical pixel size: 2–4 mm

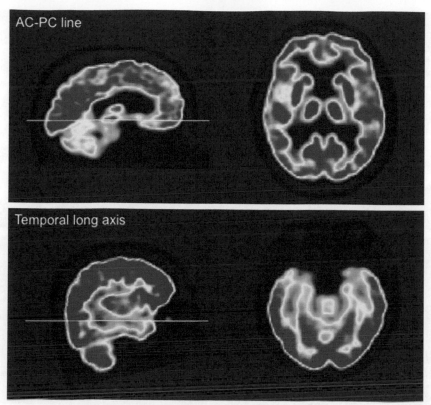

Fig. 1. 18F-FDG-PET images oriented along AC-PC line and temporal long axis.

state. For these reasons, brain shows an intense 18F-FDG uptake, with higher activity in the gray matter compared with the white matter.

In resting conditions, cerebral metabolic rate values for glucose are approximately 15 μmol/min/100 g for the white matter, and 40 to 60 μmol/min/100 g for the gray matter. In the normal brain, the gray/white matter activity ratio ranges from 2.5 to 4.1.

Differences of 18F-FDG distribution have been observed among different brain regions. 18F-FDG uptake is usually higher in the frontal, parietal, and occipital areas than in the temporal cortex, and the basal ganglia have slightly higher activity than the cortex.[9] Moreover, focal areas of increased uptake were observed in frontal eye fields, posterior cingulate cortex, and visual cortex of normal subjects. Metabolic activity is lower in medial temporal cortex, including hippocampal areas, than in neocortical regions (**Box 4, Fig. 2**).[9,10]

Brain 18F-FDG uptake is usually homogeneous and symmetric. Slight asymmetries in 18F-FDG uptake have been observed in the Wernicke area, the frontal eye fields, and the angular gyrus, with a prevalence that is generally less than 10%.[11]

IMAGING FINDINGS

Several 18F-FDG-PET studies have investigated the normal variants of brain metabolic activity. Subtle differences in cerebral metabolic activity have been observed among cognitively normal, healthy individuals, mostly as related to the effects of scanning time, age, and gender but also to the effect of medications and therapy procedures.

Scanning Time

Regional 18F-FDG uptake differences were observed in the normal human brain depending

| Box 4 |
Normal pattern of uptake
Areas of higher uptake
• Basal ganglia
• Frontal eye fields
• Posterior cingulate cortex
• Visual cortex
Areas of lower metabolic activity
• Medial temporal cortex

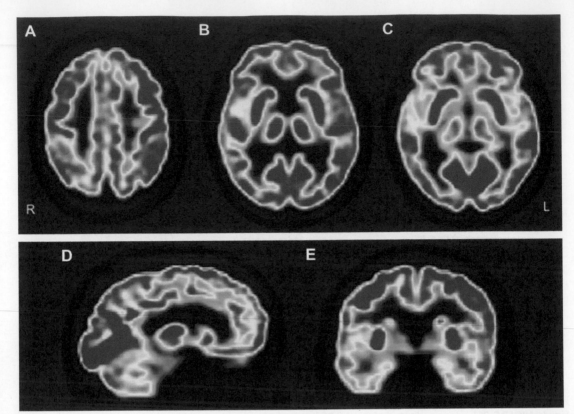

Fig. 2. 18F-FDG-PET of a normal subject. (*A–C*) Transaxial plane, showing higher 18F-FDG uptake in basal ganglia, frontal eye fields, posterior cingulate, and visual cortices. (*D*) Sagittal plane. (*E*) Coronal plane, showing lower 18F-FDG activity in temporal lobes, particularly in medial temporal cortex, compared with the other regions.

on scanning starting time after intravenous tracer injection.

Some studies compared 18F-FDG images obtained at 60 minutes after injection with earlier time frames (30 minutes after injection) in the same individuals, and showed higher 18F-FDG uptake in bilateral posterior cingulate gyrus, parietal and frontal association cortices, and subcallosal cortices, and lower uptake in cerebellum and orbitofrontal areas in scans 60 minutes after injection compared with earlier images.[12] Although the cause of such effects remains unclear, this might be because of regional differences in 18F-FDG transportation from plasma to tissue, or in glucose phosphorylation or dephosphorylation kinetics in different regions over time.[13]

Age

After the early phases of development, the human brain experiences several structural and functional changes.

According to the few 18F-FDG-PET studies on brain maturation in children, the global cerebral metabolic rate of glucose is low in the newborn period (13–25 µmol/min/100 g), and rapidly increases to adult normal values (19–33 µmol/min/100 g) at 2 years of age.[14] Global cerebral metabolic activity continues to increase to values of 49 to 65 µmol/min/100 g by age 3 to 4 years, and remains stable until approximately 9 years, when it begins to decline, reaching characteristic adult values by the end of the second decade of life.[14] This time course of global cerebral metabolic rate of glucose during childhood has been matched with the process of initial overproduction and subsequent elimination of excessive neurons and synapses occurring in the developing brain.

In addition to changes in global cerebral metabolic activity, normal brain development is associated with changes in metabolic patterns. In neonates, local cerebral glucose metabolism is highest in primitive areas, such as brainstem, cerebellar vermis, thalamus, and primary sensorimotor cortex.[14,15] Glucose metabolism in parietal, temporal (including mesial temporal region), and occipital cortices and basal ganglia increases at 3 to 5 months of age.[14,15]

In addition, the frontal cortex becomes metabolically active between 6 and 8 months.[14,15]

Although knowledge of brain metabolic changes in childhood is mainly derived from a few studies, there are more numerous 18F-FDG-PET studies of effect of age on normal adult cerebral metabolic rate of glucose.

During aging, the brain undergoes both structural and functional changes, whose regional distribution mirrors the reported cognitive decline usually observed in the normal elderly population.[16]

Enlargement of the ventricles and cortical sulci, caused by brain atrophic alterations, is one of the major changes that may occur in middle-aged to old healthy individuals. This age-related enlargement of cerebrospinal fluid spaces is reflected in brain metabolic reduction in the vicinity of ventricles, in frontobasal and perisylvian structures on 18F-FDG-PET.[17] Because these structures are mostly surrounded by white matter, their age-related hypometabolism is most likely caused by white matter atrophy occurring in healthy aging.

Besides white matter changes, healthy aging is associated with gray matter alterations.

Global cerebral metabolic rates of glucose inversely correlate with age, with a reported decline of 12–13% between the ages of 20 and 70 years.[18–20]

In addition to the global decrease in brain metabolism, several studies have reported specific patterns of age-related regional metabolic declines.

The most common metabolic reductions with advancing age have been observed in the frontal lobes (**Fig. 3**). In particular, the reduction of 18F-FDG uptake involves anterior cingulate cortex, dorsolateral and medial prefrontal cortices, and orbitofrontal cortex, bilaterally.[17,19–28] The

metabolic reduction in medial prefrontal cortices is correlated with age-associated cognitive decline in healthy subjects.[28]

Age-related metabolic decreases have also been observed in neocortical regions other than the frontal cortex, such as the insula,[20,24] the temporal lobes (particularly the temporal pole and lateral temporal cortex),[19,22,24] and the parietal lobes (including supramarginal, superior, and inferior parietal cortices).[19,20,24]

In contrast, several cortical and subcortical areas have been reported to be less affected during aging, including primary motor cortices, occipital cortices (particularly visual areas and posterior cingulate cortex), precuneus, mesial temporal lobes (hippocampus, amygdala, and parahippocampal gyrus), thalamus, putamen, pallidum, and cerebellum.[17,19,20,24,27,29] Age-related metabolic changes in healthy individuals are summarized in **Box 5**.

Brain metabolic changes observed in normal aging support the developmental theory, according to which age-related brain changes follow the phylogenetic and ontogenetic axes.[30] The topographic pattern of metabolic decline in normal aging matches, in a reverse sense, the metabolic functional changes observed in the developing human brain. The first structures to develop neurally are the same areas that are spared from metabolic deterioration occurring with age (ie, brainstem, thalamus, cerebellum, sensorimotor cortex, hippocampus), whereas the frontal regions, which become metabolically active during the third and last levels of development of the central nervous system, are the most consistently affected by the aging process.

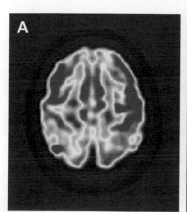
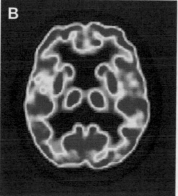
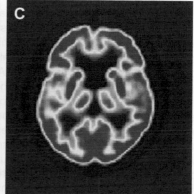

Fig. 3. Age-related metabolic reductions in 3 cognitively normal subjects. (*A*) An 80-year-old patient, showing prefrontal and superior parietal hypometabolism with sparing of primary sensorimotor cortices. (*B*) A 76-year-old patient, showing mild hypometabolism in anterior cingulate cortex, medial frontal regions, and insula. (*C*) An 82-year-old patient showing hypometabolism involving anterior cingulate cortex, medial frontal regions, and insula.

Box 5
Age-related metabolic changes in healthy individuals

Age-related hypometabolism
Frontal lobes
- Anterior cingulate cortex
- Dorsolateral and medial prefrontal cortices
- Orbitofrontal cortex

Insula
Temporal lobes
- Temporal pole
- Lateral temporal cortex

Parietal lobes
- Supramarginal, superior, and inferior parietal cortices

Least altered regions during aging
Primary motor cortices
Occipital cortices
- Visual areas
- Posterior cingulate cortex

Precuneus
Mesial temporal lobes
- Hippocampus
- Amygdala
- Parahippocampal gyrus

Thalamus
Putamen, pallidum
Cerebellum

The regional distribution of age-related hypometabolism, which primarily involves the frontal lobes, is substantially different from the patterns of brain metabolic impairment typical of Alzheimer disease (AD) and other dementias. AD is characterized by hypometabolism in precuneus and posterior cingulate cortex, parietotemporal regions, and, more variably, medial temporal regions, whereas the frontal cortex becomes affected at late disease stages.[6,31] Because many aging individuals experience memory loss, such metabolic differences make 18F-FDG-PET particularly useful in the diagnosis of AD versus normal aging, and in the understanding of age-related versus AD-related memory impairment. Although memory impairment caused by AD is linked to posterior cingulate and hippocampal hypometabolism, memory deficits observed during normal aging may reflect mainly a failure of encoding and retrieval processes of episodic memory, which depends on frontal cortex integrity.[32]

The identification of brain metabolic abnormalities typical of AD in 18F-FDG-PET of cognitively normal subjects has a strong predictive value for future development of AD. Longitudinal 18F-FDG-PET studies in normal individuals who later deteriorated to AD showed that AD-related metabolic reductions precede the onset of clinical symptoms by many years and correlate with diagnosis of AD.[33] Hippocampal metabolic impairment usually precedes that in the cortical regions in cognitively normal individuals deteriorating to dementia caused by AD, whereas the cortical hypometabolism becomes evident later.[33]

Gender

Several 18F-FDG-PET studies focused on the effect of gender on brain metabolism to highlight possible metabolic differences and corresponding behavioral differences between men and women.

Brain volume is reportedly greater in men than in women, with a higher percentage of gray matter in female and a higher percentage of white matter in male subjects.[34] However, 18F-FDG findings have been controversial, as summarized in Table 1.

The inconsistencies among studies are likely caused by differences in sample size, subjects' ages, and image analysis procedures. Hormones (eg, estrogen) are another potential source of variation in cerebral metabolism of female subjects.[35] Correction, or lack of correction, for differences in brain size and skull thickness between genders is another potential confounding factor that should be taken into account.[36]

Substances/Medications

Several substances and medications may influence the cerebral metabolic rate of glucose, predominantly altering global metabolism but also with possible effects on regional distribution (Box 6).

Among the substances capable of altering cerebral metabolism, caffeine is one of the most commonly used. Caffeine is part of the methylxanthine family and has a vasoconstrictive effect. Caffeine assumption before PET examination decreases global cerebral glucose metabolism as measured with 18F-FDG, with a mean change of -18%; the reduction is particularly prominent in the anterior cingulate cortex.[44]

Alcohol has a broad range of actions on many neurotransmitter systems. The brain metabolic response to acute administration of ethanol in

Table 1
Summary of literature on the effect of gender on cerebral glucose metabolism in normal healthy subjects

Study	M/W	Mean Age, M/W (y)	18F-FDG-PET Findings
Hsieh et al,[21] 2012	50/50	58.58/57.56	M>W in bilateral visual cortices and cerebellum
Kim et al,[22] 2009	32/46	46.6/40.6	No differences M: gender-specific age-related hypometabolism in insula W: gender-specific age-related hypometabolism in caudate nucleus
Brickman et al,[29] 2003	35/35	54.0 (all subjects)	M>W in caudate nucleus
Kawachi et al,[37] 2002	22/22	63.0/63.1	M>W in insula, middle temporal gyrus, medial frontal lobe W>M in hypothalamus
Willis et al,[20] 2002	38/28	38.1/41.0	W>M (global) W: maximal age-related hypometabolism in midsuperior temporal gyrus M: maximal age-related hypometabolism in a more superior temporal gyrus
Volkow et al,[38] 1997	15/13	44/44	W>M in temporal poles and cerebellum
Murphy et al,[39] 1996	55/65	53 (all subjects)	W>M in thalamus M>W in hippocampus
Gur et al,[40] 1995	37/24	27 (all subjects)	M>W in orbitofrontal lobes, temporal poles, temporo-occipital areas, hippocampus, and amygdala
Andreason et al,[11] 1994	21/18	26 (all subjects)	W>M in orbitofrontal and medial frontal cortices, posterior cingulate cortex, and caudate nucleus
Miura et al,[36] 1990	17/15	30 (all subjects)	No differences
Yoshii et al,[42] 1988	39/37	54 (all subjects)	W>M (global)
Baxter et al,[43] 1987	7/7	32 (all subjects)	W>M (global)

Abbreviations: M, men; W, women.
Data from Refs.[20–22,29,36–43]

healthy subjects has been investigated in several studies and it has consistently shown a global reduction of brain glucose metabolism after ethanol administration, although with various degrees across different studies (from -9% to -25%).[45–47] Discrepancies in the amount of metabolic reduction could be caused by differences in the amount of ethanol administered, PET scanners, composition of samples, and data analyses. The greatest metabolic decrease in absolute metabolism usually occurs in the occipital cortex and in the cerebellum. Moderate hypometabolism has been observed in the limbic system, parietal cortex, frontal cortex, cingulate gyrus, temporal cortex, thalamus, and midbrain. The smallest decrease has been observed in the basal ganglia.[45–47]

Abused substances such as amphetamines and cocaine significantly alter glucose brain metabolism. Low doses of amphetamines affect cerebral metabolism by decreasing metabolic rates of glucose of cortical and subcortical areas.[48] In contrast, at high doses amphetamines increase whole-brain glucose metabolism, particularly in striata, thalami, and anterior cingulate cortex.[49] Amphetamine abuse also exerts long-term effects on the brain: 18F-FDG-PET of ecstasy abusers, even after detoxification, shows hypometabolism in striata, amygdala, hippocampus, and cingulate cortex.[50]

Cocaine use before 18F-FDG-PET examination induces a significant increase of brain metabolism in several cortical and subcortical areas, directly related to the substance exposure.[51] Cocaine-induced increases in brain metabolism are localized in the medial prefrontal cortex in cases of limited exposure. As cocaine exposure increases, hypermetabolism could be observed in the prefrontal and anterior cingulate cortices and in regions of sensorimotor processing. Enhanced

Box 6
Effects of several substances and medications on cerebral glucose metabolism in normal individuals

Substance/Medication	Effect on Brain Glucose Metabolism
Caffeine	Global mean reduction (-18%), most prominent in anterior cingulate cortex
Alcohol	Global mean reduction (from -9% to -25%), most prominent in occipital cortex and cerebellum
Amphetamines	Low doses: metabolic decrease in cortical and subcortical areas
	High doses: global metabolic increase, in particular in caudate nucleus, thalamus, and anterior cingulate cortex
	Long-term effect: metabolic reduction in cingulate cortex, striata, amygdala, and hippocampus
Cocaine	Acute: increased metabolic activity in medial prefrontal cortex, expanding in prefrontal, sensorimotor, anterior cingulate cortices, and in striata
	Long term: reduced metabolic activity in striata and orbitofrontal cortex
Anesthetics	Global mean reduction (-46%)
Benzodiazepines	Global metabolic reduction, most prominent in occipitocerebellar regions
Neuroleptics	Metabolic increase in striata and thalamus
	Metabolic decrease in frontal and anterior cingulate cortices
Corticosteroids	Generalized reduction of glucose metabolic activity
Chemotherapy	Reduction in cortical metabolic activity (-17%)
	Metabolic decrease in inferior frontal cortex

Data from Refs.[44–62]

metabolic activity may be also found in the striatum.[51] In addition, 18F-FDG-PET scans of detoxified cocaine abusers may show alterations of glucose brain metabolism, with significant reduction of metabolic activity in striata and orbitofrontal cortex.[52]

Among the medications that have been shown to alter brain glucose metabolism are several drugs acting on the central nervous system, such as anesthetics, sedatives, and neuroleptics, as well as corticosteroids and chemotherapy agents.

Anesthetics, such as propofol, isoflurane, and barbiturates, produce a global, substantially uniform, metabolic reduction, at levels reaching -46% of normal metabolic activity.[53,54]

Benzodiazepines such as lorazepam induce a significant decrease in global cerebral metabolism, with more prominent reduction in the occipital cortex and cerebellum.[55]

Neuroleptic drugs such as haloperidol have been shown to increase metabolic activity in striata and thalami and to reduce glucose metabolism in the frontal lobes and anterior cingulate cortex.[56]

Moreover, consumption of corticosteroids before 18F-FDG-PET scan induces alterations of cerebral metabolism, with a generalized reduction of glucose metabolic activity.[57]

In addition, brain 18F-FDG-PET scan in cognitively normal subjects may show a lower brain metabolism (at levels around -17%) after chemotherapy than before the treatment.[58] This condition, known as chemo-brain, could also be observed years after the chemotherapy, with reduction of cortical metabolism, particularly in inferior frontal gyrus.[59,60]

Therapy Procedures

Changes occurring after radiotherapy, especially external beam radiotherapy, may mimic hypometabolism because of neurodegeneration.

In the first weeks immediately after radiotherapy, radiation may induce increased 18F-FDG uptake in normal brain tissues, caused by inflammatory changes.[63,64] These posttherapy changes could also be visible in the epithelial surfaces.

A long-term consequence after radiotherapy may be a reduction of up to -5% of cerebral metabolic activity in the irradiated brain tissue, compared with nonirradiated brain tissue.[65]

ARTIFACTS

The main factors that can cause artifacts on 18F-FDG-PET images, potentially leading to interpretation errors, are the following:

- Hyperglycemia. As 18F-FDG enters and is metabolized in cells using the same mechanisms as glucose, increased plasma glucose levels result in decreased uptake of 18F-FDG in normal brain tissue.[66] In particular, hyperglycemia can induce a reduction of 18F-FDG uptake in all brain regions (including cortical and subcortical gray matter, white matter, and cerebellum), at levels reaching -54%.[67]

- Patient motion. Patient motion during PET scanning introduces errors in the attenuation correction and image blurring leading to artifactual changes in activity concentrations and degradation of image resolution. A mismatch of as little as 5 mm may cause an error of as much as 10% in measured 18F-FDG-PET activity, and a 10-mm mismatch can cause a 25% error.[68,69] Lateral movements of the patient's head during image acquisition cause a common motion artifact showing unilateral cerebral hypometabolism, also involving the ipsilateral scalp. In these cases, non–attenuation-corrected PET images should be observed, showing the displacement of the patient's head. These artifacts can be corrected using computer realignment or calculating the attenuation correction with a standard attenuation coefficient.

- Calculated attenuation. When a transmission image or a computed tomography (CT) scan is not available, attenuation correction could be calculated using a standard attenuation coefficient. However, this method does not take into account differences across subjects, in particular variations of skull thickness. For example, subjects with hyperostosis frontalis may show artifactual reduction of frontal metabolic activity.

- Metallic artifacts. The CT-based correction method overestimates the attenuation of metallic objects included in the field of view and results in artifactually increased 18F-FDG activity in PET images. When metallic artifacts are suspected, the absence of high activity in uncorrected images should be confirmed, in order to prevent potential misinterpretation.

SUMMARY

Brain 18F-FDG-PET allows the in vivo study of cerebral glucose metabolism, reflecting neuronal and synaptic activity.

18F-FDG-PET has been extensively used to detect metabolic alterations in several neurologic diseases compared with normal aging. However, healthy subjects show variants of 18F-FDG distribution, especially as associated with aging.

In normal healthy subjects, cerebral metabolic rate values for glucose are around 15 µmol/min/ 100 g for the white matter, and around 40 to 60 µmol/min/100 g for the gray matter. 18F-FDG uptake is usually homogeneous and symmetric, but areas of slightly higher activity are observed in basal ganglia, frontal eye fields, posterior cingulate cortex, and visual cortex. In contrast, lower metabolic activity is observed in the medial temporal cortex.

During aging, the global cerebral metabolic rate of glucose decreases, with a reported decline of 12–13% between the ages of 20 and 70 years. Healthy aging is associated with mild cortical hypometabolism preferentially involving the frontal lobes, in particular the anterior cingulate cortex, dorsolateral and medial prefrontal cortices, and orbitofrontal cortex.

Age-related metabolic reductions are also observed in the insula, the temporal lobes (particularly the temporal pole and lateral temporal cortex) and the parietal lobes. Primary motor cortices, occipital cortices (particularly visual areas and posterior cingulate cortex), precuneus, mesial temporal lobes (hippocampus, amygdala and parahippocampal gyrus), thalamus, putamen, pallidum and cerebellum are the least age-affected regions.

Gender-related differences have been reported, although definitive results remain to be established.

18F-FDG uptake in the normal brain could be affected by several substances and medications, including caffeine, alcohol, abused drugs such as amphetamines and cocaine, sedatives, neuroleptics, corticosteroids, and chemotherapy agents. In addition, radiotherapy can have both short-term and long-term effects on brain metabolism, causing 18F-FDG uptake changes in irradiated brain tissue.

In addition, several artifacts may influence 18F-FDG brain distribution and cause interpretation errors.

REFERENCES

1. Sokoloff L, Reivich M, Kennedy C, et al. The [14C] deoxyglucose method for the measurement of local cerebral glucose utilization: theory, procedure, and normal values in the conscious and anesthetized albino rat. J Neurochem 1977;28:897–916.

2. Sokoloff L. Localization of functional activity in the central nervous system by measurement of glucose utilization with radioactive deoxyglucose. J Cereb Blood Flow Metab 1981;1(1):7–36. http://dx.doi.org/10.1038/jcbfm.1981.4.

3. Kennedy C, Rosiers Des MH, Sakurada O, et al. Metabolic mapping of the primary visual system of the monkey by means of the autoradiographic

[14C]deoxyglucose technique. Proc Natl Acad Sci U S A 1976;73(11):4230–4.

4. Sokoloff L. Energetics of functional activation in neural tissues. Neurochem Res 1999;24(2):321–9.

5. Shulman RG, Rothman DL, Behar KL, et al. Energetic basis of brain activity: implications for neuroimaging. Trends Neurosci 2004;27(8):489–95. http://dx.doi.org/10.1016/j.tins.2004.06.005.

6. Mosconi L, Tsui WH, Herholz K, et al. Multicenter standardized 18F-FDG PET diagnosis of mild cognitive impairment, Alzheimer's disease, and other dementias. J Nucl Med 2008;49(3):390–8. http://dx.doi.org/10.2967/jnumed.107.045385.

7. Silverman DH, Small GW, Chang CY, et al. Positron emission tomography in evaluation of dementia: regional brain metabolism and long-term outcome. JAMA 2001;286(17):2120–7.

8. Waxman AD, Herholz K, Lewis DH, et al. Society of nuclear medicine procedure guideline for FDG PET brain imaging. J Nucl Med 2009;1–12. Available at: http://interactive.snm.org/index.cfm?PageID=8490.

9. Kochunov P, Ramage AE, Lancaster JL, et al. Loss of cerebral white matter structural integrity tracks the gray matter metabolic decline in normal aging. Neuroimage 2009;45(1):17–28. http://dx.doi.org/10.1016/j.neuroimage.2008.11.010.

10. Ibáñez V, Pietrini P, Furey ML, et al. Resting state brain glucose metabolism is not reduced in normotensive healthy men during aging, after correction for brain atrophy. Brain Res Bull 2004;63(2):147–54. http://dx.doi.org/10.1016/j.brainresbull.2004.02.003.

11. Ivançević V, Alavi A, Souder E, et al. Regional cerebral glucose metabolism in healthy volunteers determined by fluordeoxyglucose positron emission tomography: appearance and variance in the transaxial, coronal, and sagittal planes. Clin Nucl Med 2000;25(8):596–602.

12. Ishii K, Sakamoto S, Hosaka K, et al. Variation in FDG uptakes in different regions in normal human brain as a function of the time (30 and 60 minutes) after injection of FDG. Ann Nucl Med 2002;16(4):299–301.

13. Sasaki H, Kanno I, Murakami M, et al. Tomographic mapping of kinetic rate constants in the fluorodeoxyglucose model using dynamic positron emission tomography. J Cereb Blood Flow Metab 1986;6(4):447–54. http://dx.doi.org/10.1038/jcbfm.1986.78.

14. Chugani HT, Phelps ME, Mazziotta JC. Positron emission tomography study of human brain functional development. Ann Neurol 1987;22(4):487–97. http://dx.doi.org/10.1002/ana.410220408.

15. Kinnala A, Suhonen-Polvi H, Aarimaa T, et al. Cerebral metabolic rate for glucose during the first six months of life: an FDG positron emission tomography study. Arch Dis Child Fetal Neonatal Ed 1996;74(3):F153–7. http://dx.doi.org/10.1136/fn.74.3.F153.

16. Baron JC, Godeau C. Human aging. In: Mazziotta JC, Toga A, Frackowiak RSJ, editors. Brain Mapping: The Systems. San Diego, Calif: Academic Press; 2000. p. 591–604.

17. Zuendorf G, Kerrouche N, Herholz K, et al. Efficient principal component analysis for multivariate 3D voxel-based mapping of brain functional imaging data sets as applied to FDG-PET and normal aging. Hum Brain Mapp 2002;18(1):13–21. http://dx.doi.org/10.1002/hbm.10069.

18. Bentourkia M, Bol A, Ivanoiu A, et al. Comparison of regional cerebral blood flow and glucose metabolism in the normal brain: effect of aging. J Neurol Sci 2000;181(1–2):19–28. http://dx.doi.org/10.1016/S0022-510X(00)00396-8.

19. Moeller JR, Ishikawa T, Dhawan V, et al. The metabolic topography of normal aging. J Cereb Blood Flow Metab 1996;16(3):385–98. http://dx.doi.org/10.1097/00004647-199605000-00005.

20. Willis MW, Ketter TA, Kimbrell TA, et al. Age, sex and laterality effects on cerebral glucose metabolism in healthy adults. Psychiatry Res 2002;114(1):23–37.

21. Hsieh TC, Lin WY, Ding HJ, et al. Sex- and age-related differences in brain FDG metabolism of healthy adults: an SPM analysis. J Neuroimaging 2012;22(1):21–7. http://dx.doi.org/10.1111/j.1552-6569.2010.00543.x.

22. Kim IJ, Kim SJ, Kim YK. Age- and sex-associated changes in cerebral glucose metabolism in normal healthy subjects: statistical parametric mapping analysis of F-18 fluorodeoxyglucose brain positron emission tomography. Acta Radiol 2009;50(10):1169–74. http://dx.doi.org/10.3109/02841850903258058.

23. Garraux G, Salmon E, Degueldre C, et al. Comparison of impaired subcortico-frontal metabolic networks in normal aging, subcortico-frontal dementia, and cortical frontal dementia. Neuroimage 1999;10(2):149–62. http://dx.doi.org/10.1006/nimg.1999.0463.

24. Kalpouzos G, Chételat G, Baron JC, et al. Voxel-based mapping of brain gray matter volume and glucose metabolism profiles in normal aging. Neurobiol Aging 2009;30(1):112–24. http://dx.doi.org/10.1016/j.neurobiolaging.2007.05.019.

25. Yanase D, Matsunari I, Yajima K, et al. Brain FDG PET study of normal aging in Japanese: effect of atrophy correction. Eur J Nucl Med Mol Imaging 2005;32(7):794–805. http://dx.doi.org/10.1007/s00259-005-1767-2.

26. Fujimoto T, Matsumoto T, Fujita S, et al. Changes in glucose metabolism due to aging and gender-related differences in the healthy human brain. Psychiatry Res 2008;164(1):58–72. http://dx.doi.org/10.1016/j.pscychresns.2006.12.014.

27. Herholz K, Salmon E, Perani D, et al. Discrimination between Alzheimer dementia and controls by

automated analysis of multicenter FDG PET. Neuroimage 2002;17(1):302–16.

28. Pardo JV, Lee JT, Sheikh SA, et al. Where the brain grows old: decline in anterior cingulate and medial prefrontal function with normal aging. Neuroimage 2007;35(3):1231–7. http://dx.doi.org/10.1016/j.neuroimage.2006.12.044.

29. Brickman AM, Buchsbaum MS, Shihabuddin L, et al. Striatal size, glucose metabolic rate, and verbal learning in normal aging. Brain Res Cogn Brain Res 2003;17(1):106–16. http://dx.doi.org/10.1016/S0926-6410(03)00085-5.

30. Grieve SM, Clark CR, Williams LM, et al. Preservation of limbic and paralimbic structures in aging. Hum Brain Mapp 2005;25(4):391–401. http://dx.doi.org/10.1002/hbm.20115.

31. Mosconi L, Brys M, Glodzik-Sobanska L, et al. Early detection of Alzheimer's disease using neuroimaging. Exp Gerontol 2007;42(1–2):129–38. http://dx.doi.org/10.1016/j.exger.2006.05.016.

32. Schacter DL, Savage CR, Alpert NM, et al. The role of hippocampus and frontal cortex in age-related memory changes: a PET study. Neuroreport 1996;7(6):1165.

33. Mosconi L, Mistur R, Switalski R, et al. FDG-PET changes in brain glucose metabolism from normal cognition to pathologically verified Alzheimer's disease. Eur J Nucl Med Mol Imaging 2009;36(5):811–22. http://dx.doi.org/10.1007/s00259-008-1039-z.

34. Cosgrove KP, Mazure CM, Staley JK. Evolving knowledge of sex differences in brain structure, function, and chemistry. Biol Psychiatry 2007;62(8):847–55.

35. Reiman EM, Armstrong SM, Matt KS, et al. The application of positron emission tomography to the study of the normal menstrual cycle. Hum Reprod 1996;11(12):2799–805.

36. Miura SA, Schapiro MB, Grady CL, et al. Effect of gender on glucose utilization rates in healthy humans: a positron emission tomography study. J Neurosci Res 1990;27(4):500–4. http://dx.doi.org/10.1002/jnr.490270410.

37. Kawachi T, Ishii K, Sakamoto S, et al. Gender differences in cerebral glucose metabolism: a PET study. J Neurol Sci 2002;199(1–2):79–83.

38. Volkow ND, Wang GJ, Fowler JS, et al. Gender differences in cerebellar metabolism: test-retest reproducibility. Am J Psychiatry 1997;154(1):119–21.

39. Murphy DG, DeCarli C, McIntosh AR, et al. Sex differences in human brain morphometry and metabolism: an in vivo quantitative magnetic resonance imaging and positron emission tomography study on the effect of aging. Arch Gen Psychiatry 1996;53(7):585–94. http://dx.doi.org/10.1001/archpsyc.1996.01830070031007.

40. Gur R, Mozley L, Mozley P, et al. Sex differences in regional cerebral glucose metabolism during a resting state. Science 1995;267(5197):528–31. http://dx.doi.org/10.1126/science.7824953.

41. Andreason PJ, Zametkin AJ, Guo AC, et al. Gender-related differences in regional cerebral glucose metabolism in normal volunteers. Psychiatry Res 1994;51(2):175–83. http://dx.doi.org/10.1016/0165-1781(94)90037-X.

42. Yoshii F, Barker WW, Chang JY, et al. Sensitivity of cerebral glucose metabolism to age, gender, brain volume, brain atrophy, and cerebrovascular risk factors. J Cereb Blood Flow Metab 1988;8(5):654–61. http://dx.doi.org/10.1038/jcbfm.1988.112.

43. Baxter LR, Mazziotta JC, Phelps ME, et al. Cerebral glucose metabolic rates in normal human females versus normal males. Psychiatry Res 1987;21(3):237–45.

44. Chen Y, Newberg AB, Wang J, et al. Caffeine's effects on resting-state oxygen and glucose metabolism: a combined MR and PET study. Proc Intl Soc Mag Reson Med 2009;17:794.

45. Volkow ND, Hitzemann R, Wolf AP, et al. Acute effects of ethanol on regional brain glucose metabolism and transport. Psychiatry Res 1990;35(1):39–48. http://dx.doi.org/10.1016/0925-4927(90)90007-S.

46. Volkow ND, Wang GJ, Franceschi D, et al. Low doses of alcohol substantially decrease glucose metabolism in the human brain. Neuroimage 2006;29(1):295–301.

47. Zhu W, Volkow ND, Ma Y, et al. Relationship between ethanol-induced changes in brain regional metabolism and its motor, behavioural and cognitive effects. Alcohol Alcohol 2004;39(1):53–8.

48. Wolkin A, Angrist B, Wolf A, et al. Effects of amphetamine on local cerebral metabolism in normal and schizophrenic subjects as determined by positron emission tomography. Psychopharmacology 1987;92(2):241–6. http://dx.doi.org/10.1007/BF00177923.

49. Vollenweider FX, Maguire RP, Leenders KL, et al. Effects of high amphetamine dose on mood and cerebral glucose metabolism in normal volunteers using positron emission tomography (PET). Psychiatry Res 1998;83(3):149–62. http://dx.doi.org/10.1016/S0925-4927(98)00033-X.

50. Buchert R, Obrocki J, Thomasius R, et al. Long-term effects of 'ecstasy' abuse on the human brain studied by FDG PET. Nucl Med Commun 2001;22(8):1–9. Available at: http://journals.lww.com/nuclearmedicinecomm/Fulltext/2001/08000/Long_term_effects_of__ecstasy__abuse_on_the_human.7.aspx.

51. Henry PK, Murnane KS, Votaw JR, et al. Acute brain metabolic effects of cocaine in rhesus monkeys with a history of cocaine use. Brain Imaging

Behav 2010;4(3–4):212–9. http://dx.doi.org/10.1007/s11682-010-9100-5.

52. Volkow ND, Hitzemann R, Wang GJ, et al. Long-term frontal brain metabolic changes in cocaine abusers. Synapse 1992;11(3):184–90. http://dx.doi.org/10.1002/syn.890110303.

53. Alkire MT, Haier RJ, Barker SJ, et al. Cerebral metabolism during propofol anesthesia in humans studied with positron emission tomography. Anesthesiology 1995;82(2):393.

54. Alkire MT, Haier RJ, Shah NK, et al. Positron emission tomography study of regional cerebral metabolism in humans during isoflurane anesthesia. Anesthesiology 1997;86(3):549.

55. Wang GJ, Volkow ND, Levy AV, et al. Measuring reproducibility of regional brain metabolic responses to lorazepam using statistical parametric maps. J Nucl Med 1999;40(5):715–20.

56. Holcomb HH, Cascella NG, Thaker GK, et al. Functional sites of neuroleptic drug action in the human brain: PET/FDG studies with and without haloperidol. Am J Psychiatry 1996;153(1):41–9.

57. Fulham MJ, Brunetti A, Aloj L. Decreased cerebral glucose metabolism in patients with brain tumors: an effect of corticosteroids. J Neurosurg 1995;83(4):657–64. Available at: http://dxdoiorg/103171/jns19958340657.

58. Sorokin J, Saboury B, Ahn JA, et al. Adverse functional effects of chemotherapy on whole-brain metabolism: a PET/CT quantitative analysis of FDG metabolic pattern of the "chemo-brain". Clin Nucl Med 2013;1. http://dx.doi.org/10.1097/RLU.0b013e318292aa81.

59. Silverman DH, Dy CJ, Castellon SA, et al. Altered frontocortical, cerebellar, and basal ganglia activity in adjuvant-treated breast cancer survivors 5-10 years after chemotherapy. Breast Cancer Res Treat 2007;103(3):303–11. http://dx.doi.org/10.1007/s10549-006-9380-z.

60. Simó M, Rifà-Ros X, Rodriguez-Fornells A, et al. Chemobrain: a systematic review of structural and functional neuroimaging studies. Neurosci Biobehav Rev 2013;37(8):1311–21. http://dx.doi.org/10.1016/j.neubiorev.2013.04.015.

61. Volkow ND, Kim S, Wang GJ, et al. Acute alcohol intoxication decreases glucose metabolism but increases acetate uptake in the human brain. Neuroimage 2012;64:277–83.

62. Wang GJ, Volkow ND, Franceschi D, et al. Regional brain metabolism during alcohol intoxication. Alcohol Clin Exp Res 2000;24(6):822–9.

63. Hautzel H, Müller-Gärtner HW. Early changes in fluorine-18-FDG uptake during radiotherapy. J Nucl Med 1997;38(9):1384–6.

64. Metser U, Even-Sapir E. Increased 18F-fluorodeoxyglucose uptake in benign, nonphysiologic lesions found on whole-body positron emission tomography/computed tomography (PET/CT): accumulated data from four years of experience with PET/CT. Semin Nucl Med 2007;37(3):206–22. http://dx.doi.org/10.1053/j.semnuclmed.2007.01.001.

65. Kesner AL, Lau VK, Speiser M, et al. Time-course of effects of external beam radiation on [18F]FDG uptake in healthy tissue and bone marrow. J Appl Clin Med Phys 2008;9(3):2747.

66. Ishimori T, Watanabe Y, Sakata C, et al. Effect of blood glucose level on physiological FDG uptake in the brain. J Nucl Med 2009;50(Suppl 2):134.

67. Ishizu K, Nishizawa S, Yonekura Y, et al. Effects of hyperglycemia on FDG uptake in human brain and glioma. J Nucl Med 1994;35(7):1104–9.

68. Andersson JL, Vagnhammar BE, Schneider H. Accurate attenuation correction despite movement during PET imaging. J Nucl Med 1995;36(4):670–8.

69. Huang SC, Hoffman EJ, Phelps ME, et al. Quantitation in positron emission computed tomography: 2. effects of inaccurate attenuation correction. J Comput Assist Tomogr 1979;3(6):804–14.

Head and Neck
Normal Variations and Benign Findings in FDG Positron Emission Tomography/ Computed Tomography Imaging

Liselotte Højgaard, MD, DMSCi[a],*, Anne Kiil Berthelsen, MD[b], Annika Loft, MD, PhD[b]

KEYWORDS

- Head and neck • Positron emission tomography • Computed tomography • Imaging
- Physiologic uptake • Benign tumors

KEY POINTS

- Physiologic uptake and other benign findings on positron emission tomography (PET)/computed tomography (CT) with FDG for the head and neck increase the risk of misinterpretation.
- PET/CT should be performed with diagnostic quality CT, including intravenous contrast media and with PET and CT interpreted by experts in both modalities to secure the highest quality.
- Knowledge of the anatomy in the head and neck region as well as the medical history of the patient is crucial.

INTRODUCTION

The head and neck region is typically included in every whole-body 18F-fluro-deoxyglucose (18F-FDG) positron emission tomography (PET)/ computed tomography (CT) scan.

The anatomy of the head and neck region is complicated, with many small structures close together and delicate structures. Interpretation of small lymph nodes and detection of small primary tumors are challenges.

The high physiologic FDG uptake in various benign structures, especially in the head and neck area, increases the risk of misinterpretation, and it is therefore mandatory to have knowledge about the pitfalls.

This article will guide the reader through these problems by discussing scanning procedures and normal findings as well as benign tumors with FDG PET/CT in the head and neck area.

PET/CT SCANNING PROTOCOLS

It is recommended that PET/CT is performed with diagnostic quality CT, including intravenous contrast media and with PET and CT interpreted by experts in both modalities to secure the highest quality. Time and effort should be spent on protocols for acquisition and image reconstruction. In a clinical setting, the CT part with intravenous contrast media can be used for PET attenuation correction, because the contrast media induced artifacts are rare and easy to detect.[1] In clinical trials, a standardized protocol including a noncontrast CT is often recommended, reducing the risk of measuring attenuation-caused false increased standardized uptake value (SUV) in relevant foci.

The patient should be well prepared with sufficient information about preparations and scanning procedures. FDG uptake in brown fat is a common

Disclosures: None.
[a] Department of Clinical Physiology, Nuclear Medicine & PET, Faculty of Health and Medical Sciences, Rigshospitalet, University of Copenhagen, KF 4011, Blegdamsvej 9, DK 2100, Copenhagen, Denmark; [b] Department of Clinical Physiology, Nuclear Medicine & PET, Rigshospitalet, University of Copenhagen, KF 4011, Blegdamsvej 9, DK 2100, Copenhagen, Denmark
* Corresponding author.
E-mail address: lottepet@rh.dk

PET Clin 9 (2014) 141–145
http://dx.doi.org/10.1016/j.cpet.2013.11.002
1556-8598/14/$ – see front matter © 2014 Elsevier Inc. All rights reserved.

finding in the head and neck area, especially in children and young adults, and especially during winter. Often the uptake is symmetric, but unilateral foci do occur. Fortunately, fat tissue is easily depicted on the CT scan. The fat tissue uptake can be reduced by letting the patient rest in a warm environment or tucked under warm blankets. In children this procedure is often sufficient. Adults can be prepared with a beta-blocking agent or muscle relaxing treatment (eg, diazepam) given 1 hour before the FDG injection followed by the same warm and comfortable rest period, although this procedure is still debatable.[2–4]

FDG

Patients must be fasting at least 6 hours prior to FDG injection; children need 4 hours fasting. In patients with diabetes, it is important that they are scheduled early in the morning for the first scans, and that special diabetes protocols are followed.

The recommended FDG dose is 4 MBq/kg body weight, maximum 500 MBq; children should receive 3 MBq/kg body weight until 16 years. Children older than 16 years should be dosed as adults.[5]

It is crucial that the patients are lying still and quietly between FDG injection and scan.

Activated brown fat tissue in the head and neck area can be decreased or even completely avoided by pretreatment with beta-blocking agents or diazepam.

Radiation Doses

Adults will receive approximately 5 mSv (0.019 mSv/MBq), and children will receive approximately 4 mSv[5] due to the FDG injection. The radiation dose from a whole-body CT scan of diagnostic quality is approximately 10 mSv, but the new CT scanners with iterative reconstruction possibilities can reduce the dose even further. In children, the radiation dose is approximately 1 to 4 mSv from the CT scan. So in total, the adult radiation dose for an FDG PET/CT whole-body scan with diagnostic quality CT is approximately 15 mSv, and in children, the dose is 5 to 8 mSv.

Scanning Protocol

For the diagnostic CT, it is important to have a meticulous preparation of both scan protocol and intravenous contrast media. The diagnostic CT parameters should be 80 to 120 mA, 120 to 140 kV, and 2 to 3 mm slice thickness. The patient should be positioned with the arms down and special immobilization devices for the head and neck area. It is recommended to give the intravenous contrast media with an automatic intravenous

pump. The delay must be set to show the contrast media in the head and neck region depending on the scanner characteristics. The reason for using intravenous contrast media in PET/CT is to discriminate the vessels from other structures more than to get enhancement in the tumor.

Patient Positioning

The patient must be positioned comfortably to avoid motion during scanning and should prior to this be asked to remove metal in area of scanning (eg, jewelry, piercings, or metal in clothes).

Acquisition Protocol

After the CT scan, the PET scan is performed, preferably in 3-dimensional mode, with an acquisition time of 2 to 4 minutes per bed position depending on the patient's size and weight.

Image Reconstruction

CT images are reconstructed with a 70 cm field of view (FOV) and a slice thickness of typically 2 mm. Attenuation and scatter-corrected PET data are reconstructed iteratively using a 3-dimensional attenuation weighted ordered subset expectation maximization (AW-OSEM) reconstruction including point spread function (PSF), and, if available, time of flight (TOF). The settings are 3 iterations, 21 subsets, and a 2 mm Gaussian filter. The images are reconstructed on a 336 × 336 or 400 × 400 matrix (scanner dependent) with a pixel size of 2 mm × 2 mm and a slice thickness of 3 mm.

PET/CT IMAGE INTERPRETATION

The quality of the PET/CT interpretation is increased, if it is done in collaboration with a specialist in nuclear medicine and a specialist in diagnostic radiology, and preferably done simultaneously. In some countries, physicians have competence in both nuclear medicine and radiology, and therefore can do the interpretation alone. However, 4 eyes see more than 2 eyes. Taking the overall costs of the PET/CT, including isotope, into account makes the costs of double-reading minor.

Knowledge of the anatomy in the head and neck region (Fig. 1) as well as the medical history of the patient, especially prior surgery or radiotherapy in the relevant region, is of course crucial.

PHYSIOLOGIC FDG UPTAKE

FDG is a glucose metabolism tracer; therefore physiologic uptake is seen in normal tissue as well as in malignant tumors. The degree of uptake

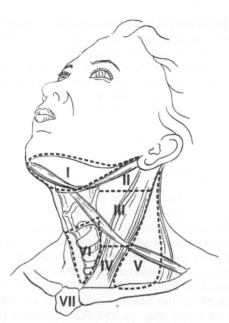

Fig. 1. Anatomy of the head and neck region. (*From* Edge SB, Byrd DR, Compton CC, et al, editors. AJCC cancer staging handbook. 6th edition. New York: Springer-Verlag; 2002. p. 29; with permission.)

(eg. measured as SUV) is not useful for discriminating between tissue types. Pattern recognition, especially with the underlying CT, is the only way to evaluate the images.

The most common sites of physiologic uptake in the head and neck region are in the salivary glands, including the sublingual glands (**Fig. 2**). These structures are most often symmetric and easy to depict on the CT scan. The degree of uptake can vary. The excretion of FDG avid saliva in the oral cavity is sometimes not symmetric and tends to be high if the patient is dehydrated.

The tonsils are always FDG avid (**Fig. 3**), and typically the uptake is symmetric. Individual variations occur, so a slight degree of asymmetry is not indicative of pathology.[6–8] In children and adolescents, lymphoid tissue of Waldeyer ring is very

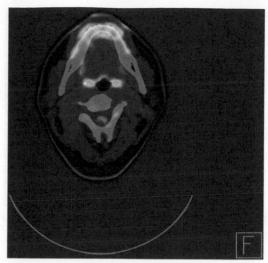

Fig. 3. High physiologic FDG uptake in the tonsils.

FDG avid; often the uptake pattern would be symmetric (**Fig. 4**).[9]

Uptake in muscular tissue is found due to contraction or previous exercise, but recent insulin injection or food intake will also give rise to high uptake. Typically this uptake is symmetric, but in case of surgery, irradiation, or muscle contraction, the pattern will be asymmetrical and much more difficult to interpret. In some areas like the paraspinal muscles, it is especially difficult (**Fig. 5**). Activity in the muscles of the tongue can be confusing, but the findings are often symmetric. Teeth grinding and chewing give rise to high muscular uptake in the mastication muscles. It is helpful to carefully examine the shape of the confusing FDG activity. Elongated shaped uptake is usually caused by physiologic uptake, whereas more focal activity tends to be pathologic. Again, the CT, especially with intravenous contrast, can be helpful in order to interpret the findings.

The vocal cords in the larynx can be FDG avid in case of speaking during the FDG uptake time. Sometimes, the uptake is unilateral and can be

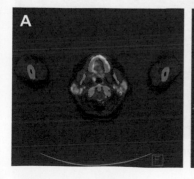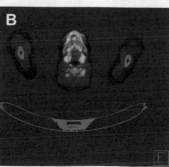

Fig. 2. (*A*) High FDG uptake in the parotid glands. (*B*) High FDG uptake in the submandibular glands.

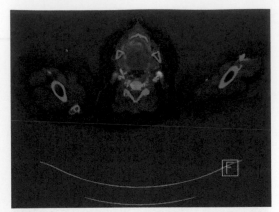

Fig. 4. FDG uptake in the lymphoid tissue of Waldeyer ring.

caused by vocal cord palsy with reduced uptake in the paralyzed cord and increased uptake in the normal cord, but the finding is not pathognomonic. Injection of calcium hydroxylapatite microspheres or other materials like Teflon used for treatment purposes can induce inflammation or even granulomatous reactions in the paralyzed cord.[10] The shape of the cord on CT is helpful for interpretation, as the paralyzed cord would be relaxed and located in the middle of the larynx.

It is important that the patient is relaxed before and during the FDG uptake period, and chewing gum should be avoided. Talking during FDG injection and uptake time should be kept at a minimum.

Diffuse uptake in the thyroid gland can be a normal variant in euthyroid patients, but hyperthyroidism and chronic thyroiditis can also be the cause. Focal uptake in the thyroid due to benign adenomas is a common finding. As 30% or more of the foci are malignant, and CT can most often not discriminate a benign finding from a malignant

one in the thyroid, a supplementary thyroid scintigraphy and/or ultrasound is recommended. Remember to postpone the thyroid scintigraphy for a minimum of 8 weeks if the PET/CT scan was performed with intravenous contrast, since the contrast contains iodine.

Physiologic uptake in the spinal cord is typically higher at the cervical level but is recognized because of the diffuse distribution.

BENIGN FINDINGS

Pleomorphic adenoma is a common benign salivary gland neoplasm characterized by neoplastic proliferation of parenchymatous glandular cells along with myoepithelial components, having a malignant potentiality. It is the most common type of salivary gland tumor and the most common tumor of the parotid gland. Warthin's tumor is also seen often, the second most common benign parotid tumor (**Fig. 6**). The FDG uptake is high, and on CT, the tumor is hyperdense and contrast media enhanced but with a characteristic well defined appearance.[10]

Inflammation caused by radiation therapy or recent surgery may give rise to increased FDG uptake diffusely in the various tissues. This kind of uptake is seldom focal and does not give rise to interpretation difficulties. However, infection can induce high uptake and can be focal as in abscesses. Oppositely, reactive uptake in lymph nodes can be difficult to discriminate from malignant metastatic spread, and malignant tissue can give rise to reactive lymph nodes. The degree of FDG uptake is not very helpful, and CT does not add diagnostic information. A full medical history is always important, but crucial in these challenging patients.

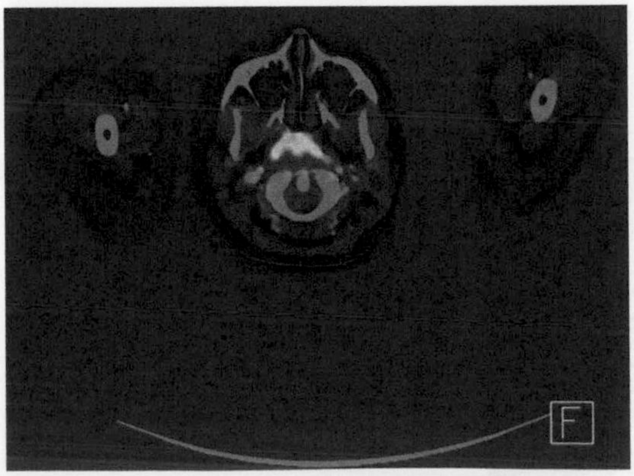

Fig. 5. Foci with high FDG uptake on the left side of the neck difficult to interpret on transaxial images.

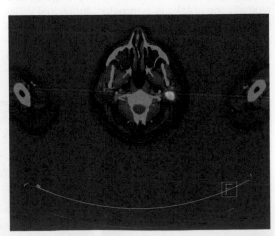

Fig. 6. High FDG uptake in a Warthin tumor in the left parotid gland.

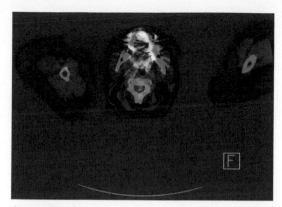

Fig. 7. Streak artifacts from teeth inducing false-positive focus.

ARTIFACTS

Artifacts in PET/CT are a well-known problem in whole-body examinations and should therefore be considered also in head and neck studies.

Metal devices, especially dental implants, give rise to streak artifacts in CT, whether acquired at low doses or of diagnostic quality. In a combined PET/CT scanner, the CT data are used for attenuation correction, and the streak artifacts will therefore induce false-positive foci (**Fig. 7**).

Beware of misalignment/misregistration of PET and CT images, as the head is more prone to motion than the rest of the body.

SUMMARY

The head and neck area is a difficult region to interpret due to many physiologic and benign findings, and it is therefore important to be aware of the many possible pitfalls.

REFERENCES

1. Berthelsen AK, Holm S, Loft A, et al. PET/CT with intravenous contrast media can be used for PET attenuation correction in cancer patients. Eur J Nucl Med Mol Imaging 2005;32:1167–75.
2. Tatsumi M, Engles JM, Ishimori T, et al. Intense (18) F-FDG uptake in brown fat can be reduced pharmacologically. J Nucl Med 2004;45:1189–93.
3. Barrington SF, Maisey MN. Skeletal muscle uptake of fluorine-18-FDG: effect of oral diazepam. J Nucl Med 1996;37:1127–9.
4. Sturkenboom MG, Hoekstra OS, Postema EJ, et al. A randomised controlled trial assessing the effect of oral diazepam on 18F-FDG uptake in the neck and upper chest region. Mol Imaging Biol 2009;11: 364–8.
5. Lassmann M, Biassoni L, Monsieurs M, et al. The new EANM paediatric dosage card. EANM Dosimetry and Paediatrics Committees. Eur J Nucl Med Mol Imaging 2008;35:1748.
6. Nakamoto Y, Tatsumi M, Hammoud D, et al. Normal FDG distribution patterns in the head and neck: PET/CT evaluation. Radiology 2005;234:879–85.
7. Bhargava P, Rahman S, Wendt J. Atlas of confounding factors in head and neck PET/CT imaging. Clin Nucl Med 2011;36:e20–9.
8. Blodgett TM, Fukui MB, Snyderman CH, et al. Combined PET-CT in the head and neck: part 1. Physiologic, altered physiologic, and artifactual FDG uptake [review]. Radiographics 2005;25:897–912.
9. Klijanienko J, Vielh P. Fine needle sampling of salivary gland lesions II. Cytology and histology correlation of 71 cases of Warthin's tumor (adenolymphoma). Diagn Cytopathol 1997;16:221–5.
10. Halpern BS, Britz-Cunningham S, Kim CK. Intense focal F-18 FDG uptake in vocal cord associated with injection of calcium hydroxylapatite microspheres. Clin Nucl Med 2011;36:e175–7.

Thorax
Normal and Benign Pathologic Patterns in FDG-PET/CT Imaging

Jason W. Wachsmann, MD[a],
Victor H. Gerbaudo, PhD, MSHCA[b],*

KEYWORDS

- Thorax • ^{18}F-Fluorodeoxyglucose PET • Computed tomography • Normal biodistribution
- Benign pathologic findings • Infection • Inflammation

KEY POINTS

- The use of ^{18}F-fluorodeoxyglucose (FDG)-PET/computed tomography (CT) for imaging of the chest has become a valuable and cost-effective tool in clinical practice.
- When relying on FDG-PET/CT imaging to characterize the nature of thoracic indeterminate findings on conventional imaging modalities, it should always be kept in mind that FDG's distribution is not limited to malignant lesions.
- Familiarity with the normal thoracic biodistribution of FDG, coupled with knowledge of the potential benign causes of increased FDG uptake in the thorax, is essential in minimizing the incidence of incorrect interpretation of FDG-PET images in daily clinical practice.

INTRODUCTION

The use of ^{18}F-fluorodeoxyglucose (FDG)-PET/computed tomography (CT) for imaging of the chest has become a very useful and cost-effective tool in daily clinical practice. The Centers for Medicare and Medicaid Services originally approved its clinical use in 1998. Thoracic malignancies were included among the first approved indications (ie, characterization of solitary pulmonary nodules and the staging of lung cancer).[1] At the time of writing, FDG-PET/CT is already an integral component of oncologic practice. Surgical and clinical oncologists rely on the information provided by FDG-PET/CT images to characterize lesions as benign or malignant, stage cancer, determine prognosis, monitor response to therapy, and assess for the presence or absence of tumor recurrence.[2,3]

The technique's success rests on its inherent ability to interrogate the biological behavior of malignant molecular pathways as opposed to just size and shape of a particular lesion. However, when relying on FDG-PET/CT to characterize the nature of suspicious findings on conventional imaging modalities, the user should keep in mind that FDG's distribution is not limited to only cancerous lesions. FDG is a structural analogue of 2-deoxyglucose and serves as a tracer of glucose metabolism, and thus as a fuel source for benign as well as malignant tissue. FDG is delivered to cells via blood flow and then enters the cell by the facilitated transport mediated by GLUT transporters. Once in the cytosol, FDG is phosphorylated by hexokinase to FDG-6-phosphate. FDG-6-phosphate is then trapped intracellularly or can be dephosphorylated back

[a] Joint Program in Nuclear Medicine, Division of Nuclear Medicine and Molecular Imaging, Department of Radiology, Brigham and Women's Hospital, Harvard Medical School, 75 Francis Street, Boston, MA 02115, USA; [b] Division of Nuclear Medicine & Molecular Imaging, Department of Radiology, Brigham & Women's Hospital and Harvard Medical School, 75 Francis Street, Boston, MA 02115, USA
* Corresponding author.
E-mail address: vgerbaudo@partners.org

PET Clin 9 (2014) 147–168
http://dx.doi.org/10.1016/j.cpet.2013.10.004
1556-8598/14/$ – see front matter © 2014 Elsevier Inc. All rights reserved.

to FDG by glucose-6-phosphatase, and reversely transported out of the cell. The latter reaction is observed in some normal tissues with high phosphatase activity, such as the liver and the resting skeletal muscle, in certain malignancies such as hepatocellular carcinomas, and in benign inflammatory cells (ie, neutrophils and macrophages). In part, this explains why benign pathologic processes, such as sterile, pyogenic, and granulomatous inflammatory lesions, take up FDG with lower, equal, or even higher intensity than malignant tissues.

Although pathologically benign chest lesions generally have a lower degree of FDG avidity in comparison with malignant lesions, there is much overlap in the intensity of uptake between them. In turn, this accounts for the difficult task to set a specific standardized uptake value (SUV) cutoff to differentiate benign from malignant disease.[4] Infection or inflammation can be highly FDG avid to the point that it may exceed the rate of hypermetabolism often observed in low-grade and, sometimes, high-grade malignancies.[5]

Familiarity with the normal thoracic biodistribution of FDG, with the variables influencing its uptake and with its behavior in benign pathologic conditions affecting the chest, is essential in interpreting FDG-PET images accurately when diagnosing, staging, and monitoring therapeutic response, and restaging cancer. This review focuses on the patterns of FDG distribution in normal and in some of the most common benign pathologic processes affecting the thorax.

PATTERNS OF FDG BIODISTRIBUTION IN THE NORMAL THORAX

The distribution of FDG in PET images of the chest can be appreciated from the skin surface peripherally to the normal physiologic activity in the mediastinal blood pool (**Fig. 1**). Cutaneous distribution of tracer is usually mild and without focality in the attenuation-corrected images of the normal patient. The skin's signal is higher on non–attenuation-corrected images secondary to the lesser amount of attenuating tissues that 511 keV coincidence photons travel through in superficial surfaces. Truncation, a common artifact on attenuation-corrected images, can be identified from the skin surface peripherally to the extent of the artifact centrally. This artifact is the result of a smaller field of view with which the CT images were acquired being applied to the PET data for attenuation correction.

Subcutaneous FDG distribution is variable based on the type of tissues being imaged. The distribution of radiotracer in the breast correlates

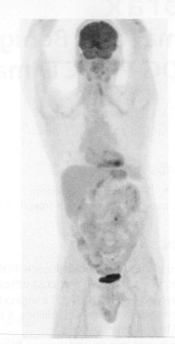

Fig. 1. Whole-body ^{18}F-fluorodeoxyglucose (FDG)-PET/computed tomography (CT) maximum-intensity projection (MIP) image showing normal physiologic distribution of FDG. Variable uptake of radiotracer is observed in the myocardium, with normal low and diffuse tracer avidity in the mediastinal blood pool. The lung parenchyma has only minimal uptake, as does the normal skeletal muscle.

with the amount of active glandular tissue (**Fig. 2**).[6] In fact this accounts for the associated increase in FDG uptake in the male patient with gynecomastia. Breast uptake varies mildly with the menstrual cycle, with the higher uptake observed in the postovulatory phase. The lactating breasts are characterized by bilateral heterogeneous and intense FDG distribution (see **Fig. 2**). FDG uptake in breast tissue decreases with increasing age and lower density.

Typically, subcutaneous adipose tissue has less tracer uptake than activated brown adipose tissue. In the thorax, uptake of brown fat may be present in the axillae, the supraclavicular and paravertebral regions, and the mediastinum (**Fig. 3**). Effective patient preparations to reduce brown adipose activation include keeping the patient warm, pharmacologic interventions such as propranolol, fentanyl, or diazepam, dietary changes, and proper temperature control in the room before and after FDG administration.[7]

Physiologic distribution of the radiotracer in the marrow of osseous structures of the chest is variable, and generally of higher intensity than the blood pool, with a typical maximum SUV (SUV$_{max}$) of less than 3.[8] Pediatric patients may have

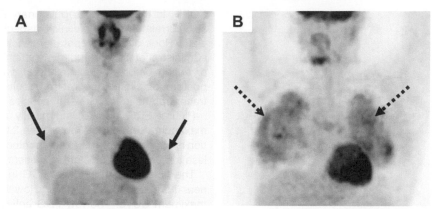

Fig. 2. FDG-PET MIP images illustrating normal patterns of FDG uptake in the breast. (*A*) Diffuse and low FDG uptake in normal breast tissue bilaterally (*solid arrows*). (*B*) Intense and heterogeneous FDG distribution is seen bilaterally in lactating breasts (*dotted arrows*).

a different pattern of tracer accumulation because of the metabolically active growth plates observed in the growing patient.[9] Marrow stimulation by growth colony stimulating factor, chemotherapy, and anemia may cause increased and diffuse radiotracer uptake in the marrow that may persist for as long as 1 year (**Fig. 4**).[8] On the other hand, photopenic areas in the marrow exposed to radiation treatment are not uncommon (**Fig. 5**). Areas of focal intense uptake are frequent in healing rib fractures and healing sternotomy (**Fig. 6**). Vertebral compression fractures treated with vertebroplasty can be highly FDG avid, and should not be confused with metastatic disease.

Muscular uptake of FDG is based on glycolytic metabolism in fast-twitch muscle fibers.[8] Uptake may be secondary to muscle contraction or may be seen in the paraspinal muscles because of the patient's anxiety.[10] Intense physical activity before the examination may lead to increased skeletal muscle uptake, with symmetry being variable (**Fig. 7**).[11] Intercostal and sometimes diaphragmatic muscle uptake is not uncommon in patients with chronic obstructive pulmonary disease (COPD) and airway obstruction (**Fig. 8**). Abnormal FDG avidity by the respiratory muscles secondary to resistance to airflow and diminished lung elasticity correlates with the severity of

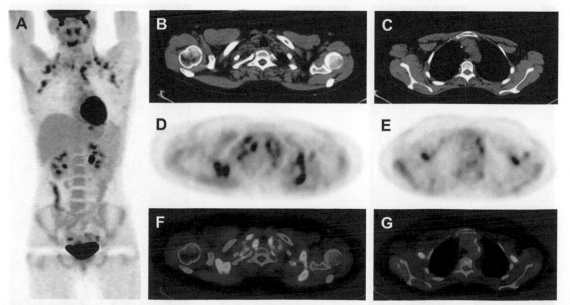

Fig. 3. (*A*) FDG-PET MIP image showing areas of increased FDG uptake in the axillary, supraclavicular, and left mediastinal areas. Transaxial FDG-PET images (*D, E*) and fused transaxial FDG-PET/CT slices (*F, G*) confirm that the regions of increased tracer avidity correspond to adipose tissue (on *B, C*). This pattern is typical of brown fat activation, and may be confused with disease in the absence of the anatomic localization image.

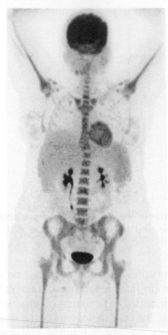

Fig. 4. Bone marrow expansion post marrow-stimulating agent in a patient with a history of lymphoma. Whole-body FDG-PET/CT MIP image shows a typical pattern of diffusely increased tracer accumulation in the axial and proximal appendicular skeleton following the administration of granulocyte colony-stimulating factor. A complete clinical and therapeutic history is helpful in distinguishing such findings from a marrow-infiltrative process.

COPD. In these patients pulmonary FDG activity also correlates with the clinical aspects of the disease. Poor patient preparation, including insulin administration before or directly after FDG infusion or eating before the examination, which causes postprandial insulin secretion, results in elevated tracer uptake in the skeletal muscles.[12]

Pleural FDG uptake is typically mild, with a maximum normal SUV lower than 2.0.[13] Distribution is normally symmetric and nonfocally avid, unless a pathologic correlate is present.

The normal distribution of FDG in the lungs is near homogeneous, with very low average and maximum SUVs. The low FDG activity observed in the aerated lung is sometimes contrasted by the greater uptake in blood vessels and bronchi at the lobar and segmental levels. Patterns of radiotracer accumulation in atelectasis can be diffuse and homogeneous, with an SUV in the low to moderate range (1.44 ± 0.54), and usually with a good correlation between the density of collapsed lung and the degree of uptake observed (**Fig. 9**).[14] In general, independent of the amount of collapsed lung, FDG uptake in atelectasis is higher than in the normal lung, but lower than in cancerous lesions.[14] The accurate differentiation between tumor and atelectasis achieved with FDG-PET has proven benefit in estimating appropriate size portals during radiation therapy

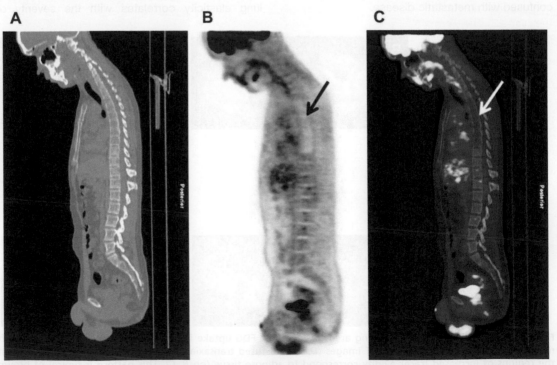

Fig. 5. (A–C) Sagittal CT, FDG-PET and fused PET/CT images, showing decreased FDG marrow uptake in thoracic vertebrae following external beam radiation for mediastinal malignancy (*arrows in B, C*).

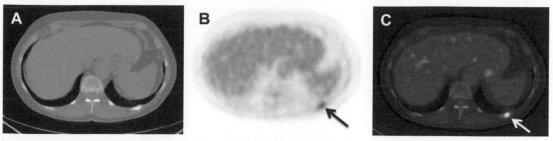

Fig. 6. Transaxial CT (*A*), FDG-PET (*B*), and fused FDG-PET/CT (*C*) images demonstrating the typical pattern of post-traumatic FDG uptake in a healing posterior left rib fracture (*arrows in B, C*).

planning, thereby to minimize radiation dose to normal tissue.

The mediastinal biodistribution of radiotracer in PET images is secondary to uptake in several structures including the thymus, vessels, heart, pericardium, esophagus, lymph nodes, blood pool, and adipose tissue. Thymic uptake can be variable based on the age of the patient. Normal thymic uptake is usually above that of the blood pool, and tends to be higher in the population younger than 30 years, with a correlation between the level of uptake and the density of the gland.[15] Thymic hyperplasia is a nonmalignant response to chemotherapy, believed to be caused by immunologic rebound and infiltration of plasma cells, and characterized by moderate FDG avidity throughout the enlarged gland (**Fig. 10**).[16] Sometimes malignant involvement can be differentiated from hyperplasia by the morphology and size of the gland.[16] The normal gland SUV_{max} has been reported to be 1.8 ± 0.55,[16] with FDG-PET/CT

not considered useful in differentiating between malignant and benign thymic tumors (**Fig. 11**).[17]

Myocardial FDG uptake is variable and depends on the state of fasting, plasma glucose, and free fatty acid and insulin levels (**Figs. 12 and 13**). In the fasting state, the myocardium preferentially uses fatty acids as its primary energy source.[18] Therefore, after a fast of approximately 4 hours, the myocardium shifts from glycolytic to fatty acid metabolism as its primary source of energy, with the subsequent reduction in FDG uptake. On the other hand, postprandially or after glucose loading the myocytes preferentially use glucose. In the fasting state the ischemic myocardium is expected to take up more FDG than do normal segments. Therefore patients are prepared with a glucose load before myocardial FDG-PET to enhance the uptake in the normal myocardium in comparison with ischemic segments. By contrast, a long fasting state (6–12 hours) is recommended for oncologic imaging, to minimize the possibility

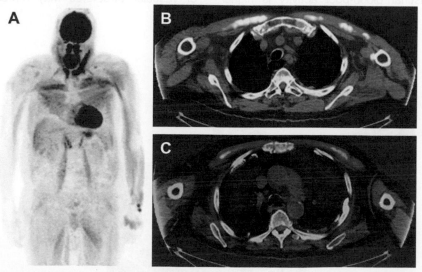

Fig. 7. Moderate and diffuse muscular FDG uptake is present most prominently in the pectoralis muscles in a patient who reported strenuous exercise before his FDG injection and imaging. (*A*) FDG-PET MIP; (*B, C*) transaxial FDG-PET/CT images at 2 different levels of the patient's chest.

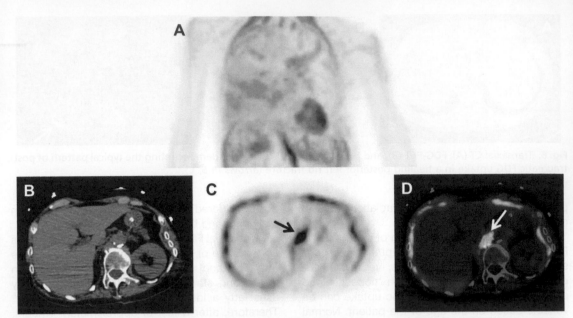

Fig. 8. (*A*) FDG-PET MIP image shows intercostal and diaphragmatic muscle uptake, confirmed in (*B*) transaxial CT, (*C*) FDG-PET, and (*D*) fused FDG-PET/CT images of a patient with chronic obstructive pulmonary disease and respiratory distress. The degree of tracer uptake in these regions has been shown to correspond to more advanced disease clinically. Note the FDG-avid right retrocrural lymph node on images *C–D* (*arrows*), in this patient with a previous history of lymphoma.

of undesired myocardial uptake obscuring malignant nodes in the mediastinum of the patient with cancer.[8,18] Pericardial uptake is uncommon in FDG-PET/CT, with benign focal pericardial thickening being usually not FDG avid.[18]

FDG uptake in the vasculature of the chest is primarily dependent on the amount of radiotracer present in the blood pool (see Figs. **1**, **2**, **12**, and **13**).[8] Mediastinal blood-pool activity is higher than lung activity in attenuation-corrected images. FDG activity in the blood pool of the lungs decreases as a function of time after injection. In general, activity in the blood pool decreases slightly over time, as FDG distributes in target tissues and is excreted by the kidneys. Therefore, blood-pool activity will be higher than expected in patients with renal failure. Normal uptake in the walls of vascular structures may represent smooth

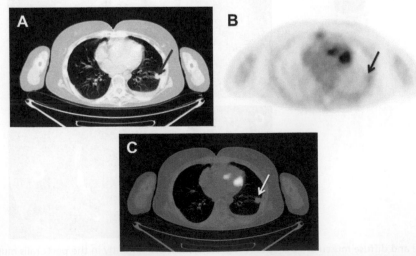

Fig. 9. (*A*) Transaxial CT slice in lung window shows rounded atelectasis in the left lung (*red arrow*), with very low FDG uptake on (*B*) transaxial FDG-PET and (*C*) fused transaxial FDG-PET/CT (*black and white arrows*, respectively).

Baseline   Post-Chemotherapy

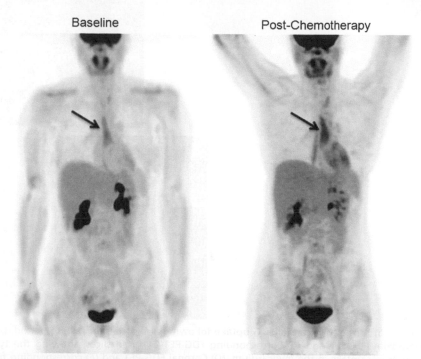

Fig. 10. (*Left*) Baseline FDG-PET MIP image shows normal thymic FDG uptake, which is typically mild and in an inverted triangular shape (*arrow*). (*Right*) Postchemotherapy image demonstrates increased intensity and size of the thymic gland (*arrow*) that has undergone rebound following treatment.

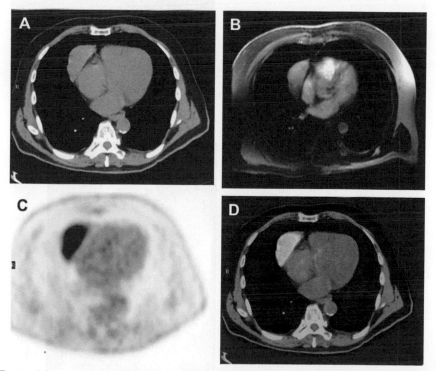

Fig. 11. (*A*) Transaxial non–contrast-enhanced CT and (*B*) transaxial contrast-enhanced T1-weighted magnetic resonance images show a soft-tissue mass along the right anteromedial aspect of the heart. (*C*) Corresponding FDG-PET and (*D*) FDG-PET/CT fusion images show diffuse and intense radiotracer uptake in the mass, which later was confirmed by biopsy as thymoma.

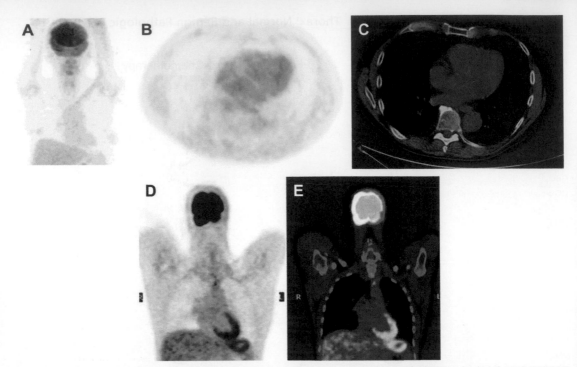

Fig. 12. Common patterns of myocardial FDG uptake following a 4- to 6-hour fasting period. (*A*) FDG-PET MIP image. (*B*) Transaxial FDG-PET and (*C*) corresponding FDG-PET/CT fused slices, showing the typically normal, diffuse, and low tracer uptake in the myocardium. (*D*) Coronal FDG-PET and (*E*) corresponding fused PET/CT images show persistent and moderate FDG uptake in the anterior, apical, and inferior walls of the left ventricle.

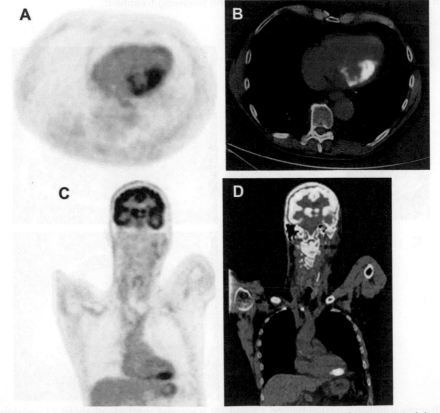

Fig. 13. Common patterns of myocardial FDG uptake following a 4- to 6-hour fasting period (continued). (*A*) Axial FDG-PET and (*B*) corresponding fused FDG-PET/CT images show variable and segmental myocardial uptake of FDG in the basal to mid-posterolateral left ventricle. (*C*) Coronal FDG-PET and (*D*) corresponding fused FDG-PET/CT images show intense and focal uptake of the radiotracer in the inferoapical wall of the left ventricle.

muscle metabolism, and/or a certain degree of subendothelial smooth muscle proliferation associated with aging.

FDG uptake is normally present in the gastrointestinal tract of the chest with variable intensity. Distal esophageal uptake near the gastroesophageal junction can be normal, and should not be presumed to represent neoplasm (**Fig. 14**). Diffuse esophageal uptake is a normal finding as well; however, when inflammation is present uptake may be more intense, and usually follows a linear pattern along the esophagus, as described in more detail later (**Fig. 15**).[19]

A wide range of normal levels of uptake in pulmonary hilar nodes has been described. The average SUV_{max} in the hilar nodes of a healthy population has been reported to be 1.1 ± 3.0, with an average CT size of 1.55 × 1.46 cm.[20] Symmetric hilar uptake on 2 consecutive FDG-PET/CT scans in patients without lung cancer is highly compatible with a benign etiology.[21]

PATTERNS OF FDG UPTAKE IN BENIGN PATHOLOGIC PROCESSES OF THE THORAX
Infection

Chest-wall infection can be the result of direct trauma, extension from adjacent soft tissues such as the lung or pleura, or even the result of

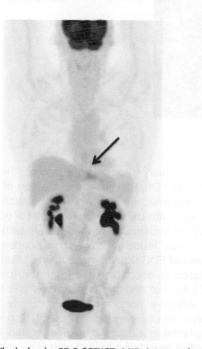

Fig. 14. Whole-body FDG-PET/CT MIP image shows mild to moderate normal tracer accumulation at the gastroesophageal junction (*arrow*). It is important that this is recognized as physiologic, to prevent further invasive procedures such as endoscopy.

osteomyelitis with local extension. Primary chest-wall infection is rare, but can be seen in patients with diabetes mellitus or the immunosuppressed.[22] FDG uptake in infectious processes results from tracer accumulation in the inflammatory immune response to the process, more so than in the organism causing the infection. Uptake in the activated immune cells is secondary to the fact that they express active glucose transporters and hexokinase. Affinity for glucose is also increased in the responding immune cells secondary to cytokines and growth factors.[23] The most common etiologic factor of pyogenic infection of the chest wall, more specifically osteomyelitis of the rib cage, is *Staphylococcus aureus*.[24] Tuberculosis is an uncommon source of chest-wall infection, but may occur following spread from adjacent tissues or hematogenous spread. Actinomycosis is also a rare cause of bacterial chest-wall infection, but is known to cause FDG-avid fistulas involving the chest wall and pleura, resulting from the damaging activity of its proteolytic enzymes.[22]

Osteomyelitis, an infection of the bone and bone marrow, is most commonly caused by bacteria and mycobacteria. It is typically the result of hematogenous spread, direct inoculation, or extension from adjacent soft tissues. Hematogenous spread of infection is more common In children, whereas spread of infection secondary to contiguous foci accounts for more than half of osteomyelitis cases in adults.[25,26,27] FDG uptake in normal cortical bone is low, with more variable uptake in marrow. Thus, the increased tracer accumulation associated with bone infection places FDG-PET at an advantage for its detection and characterization.[23] A systematic review and meta-analysis of the literature showed that when compared with other modalities, FDG-PET had the highest diagnostic accuracy in confirming or excluding osteomyelitis, especially in the axial skeleton.[26] Sensitivity of 96% for FDG-PET was significantly superior to 82% for bone scintigraphy, 61% for leukocyte scintigraphy, 78% for combined bone and leukocyte scintigraphy, and 84% for magnetic resonance imaging. FDG-PET also had the highest specificity of 91% in comparison with the other modalities.[26]

Infection of the lung parenchyma can be caused by several organisms, such as typical bacteria, mycobacteria, and viral and fungal organisms. In addition, other clinical entities, such as aspiration of gastric contents or chemical agents, can be the cause of infection.[28] Pulmonary infection can be falsely interpreted as tumor in FDG-PET, given the increased glycolysis observed in the cell-mediated inflammatory response with associated increased FDG metabolism (**Fig. 16**).[29] FDG-PET

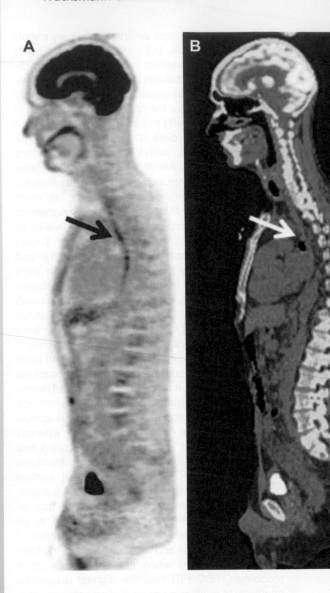

A

B

Fig. 15. (A) Sagittal FDG-PET and (B) corresponding fused FDG-PET/CT images show a linear pattern of moderate FDG avidity along the thoracic esophagus (*arrow*) in a patient with known radiation-induced esophagitis.

imaging cannot characterize reliably the pathogen of the infection based on intensity or pattern of uptake, because most of the tracer is taken up by the inflammatory cells rather than the pathogen.[23]

The most common cause of mediastinal infection is direct invasion following surgical intervention. However, just as for infection elsewhere, direct extension from adjacent disease and hematogenous spread to the mediastinum is also possible. Mediastinal infection is classified as acute or chronic, and is associated with high morbidity and mortality.[30] The utility of FDG-PET has not been evaluated in a controlled study as yet, and given that postoperative change is the most common cause of mediastinal infection, the technique plays a limited role.

Preliminary reports have shown the potential value of FDG-PET for the evaluation of infectious endocarditis. In a study of patients with infectious endocarditis using the Duke criteria of echocardiographic findings, all of the patients with the infection were found to have corresponding elevated levels of FDG uptake in the heart.[31] Further investigation is needed to elucidate the role of FDG-PET/CT not only in the diagnosis and monitoring of infective endocarditis, particularly prosthetic valve infective endocarditis, but also in cardiac implantable electronic device–related infections. A case report of a patient with FDG-avid tuberculous constrictive pericarditis showed that PET may play an important clinical role by being able to assess response to treatment in its early phase.[32] Increased and mildly heterogeneous FDG uptake

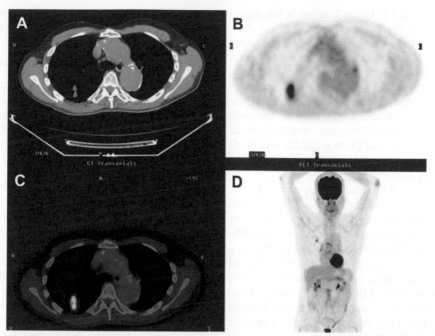

Fig. 16. A 45-year-old male smoker from the Ohio River valley with a solitary pulmonary nodule undergoing PET/CT imaging for lesion characterization. (*A*) Transaxial noncontrast CT image shows soft-tissue density in the posterior right lung, which is intensely FDG avid in (*B*) axial FDG-PET, (*C*) fused FDG-PET/CT, and (*D*) FDG-PET MIP images. It is important to always keep nonmalignant etiologic factors on the differential diagnosis, as this pathologically proven case of histoplasmosis could be easily mistaken for malignancy In this patient with a high pretest probability of lung malignancy.

in the ventricular wall of a patient with biopsy-proven Epstein-Barr viral myocarditis has also been reported.[33]

Interstitial Lung Disease, Connective Tissue Disease, and Vasculitides

There is a broad category of chest diseases that can be characterized as "other." In this article the category includes interstitial lung disease, connective tissue disease, and others that are somewhat difficult to characterize.

Interstitial lung disease consists of a large group of disorders with variable causes, treatments, and prognoses. These disorders are typically grouped according to their similar clinical distribution and are based on the findings on conventional chest films. Dyspnea and nonproductive cough are the most common symptoms at presentation. Although there is variability in the specific patterns of findings on chest radiography, there is generally volume loss with reticular or reticulonodular opacities. Typically patients present with a restrictive pattern in pulmonary function tests and decreased CO_2 diffusion capacity. Causes include occupational exposure, medical exposure, hypersensitivity, collagen vascular disease, or idiopathic etiology.[34]

In a study of 36 consecutive patients analyzing the intensity of FDG uptake in interstitial pulmonary fibrosis and diffuse parenchymal lung disease, the investigators showed that radiotracer uptake was increased to more than twice that in normal lung in areas of diseased lung.[35] In addition, the mean mediastinal lymph node uptake was found to correlate significantly with pulmonary avidity for FDG. There was also a good correlation between FDG uptake and lung function. Follow-up imaging showed that in most of these patients, the areas with higher tracer accumulation subsequently went on to develop corresponding honeycombing on high-resolution lung CT. This study highlights that the necessity and timing of therapeutic intervention can be determined based on the FDG-PET results. However, this study also showed that interstitial pulmonary fibrosis could not be differentiated from other causes of diffuse parenchymal lung disease based on FDG uptake values alone.[35] The mechanism responsible for increased FDG metabolism in interstitial lung disease is not clear at the time of writing, but typically there is increased tracer uptake by the inflammatory immune response across disease entities. Considering that fibroblasts are the primary mediators in all of the proposed models of pathogenesis of the disease, it is probably safe to postulate that what is being imaged is the actual metabolism of activated fibroblasts.[35]

Connective tissue–associated interstitial lung disease is a common complication mostly seen in immunologic disorders such as scleroderma, rheumatoid arthritis, Sjögren syndrome, polymyositis, dermatomyositis, and systemic lupus erythematosus. There is poor correlation between pulmonary and nonpulmonary manifestations, with some evidence that there is diffuse and moderate FDG uptake in connective tissue–associated interstitial lung disease.[36]

The most common pulmonary vasculitides, such as Wegener granulomatosis, microscopic polyangiitis, and Churg-Strauss syndrome, are associated with antineutrophil cytoplasmic antibodies. Cellular inflammation, vessel destruction, and necrosis are the pathologic hallmarks of vasculitis, which have been shown to be FDG avid.[23,37] Therefore, FDG-PET/CT could prove useful for evaluating activity in these lesions, determining the most adequate biopsy site, and therapeutic monitoring and follow-up.

Pneumoconiosis

Pneumoconiosis includes a group of inhalation-related restrictive lung diseases that are typically work related. The name of the disease is related to the type of material inhaled, such as asbestosis, silicosis, berylliosis, or coal-related disease. Variable degrees of FDG uptake have been described both in the pulmonary findings and in nonmalignant mediastinal and/or hilar lymph nodes.[38,39,40] In cases of pneumoconiosis the SUV in parenchymal lesions can reach intensities typically seen in malignant nodules.[38] In silicosis, peripherally diffuse and intense FDG uptake in both lungs, coupled with low tracer activity in the mediastinal lymph nodes, is usually consistent with areas of active inflammation.[40] Considering the pro-oncogenic properties of pneumoconiosis, the similarity in intensity and patterns of FDG uptake between these lesions and cancer can become an undesirable source of false-positive results.

Acute Respiratory Distress Syndrome

Acute respiratory distress syndrome is characterized pathologically by diffuse damage to the alveolar capillary walls, increased capillary permeability, pulmonary edema, neutrophil and macrophage infiltration with fibrin exudation, and hyaline membrane formation. Increased FDG uptake has been described by various investigators, and consists of a diffuse pattern of increased uptake in areas of airspace disease.[41,42] In fact, acute respiratory distress syndrome can be differentiated from pulmonary contusion based on the typical diffuse distribution of the former.[42]

Treatment-Related Sources of Abnormal FDG Uptake

Several treatment-related causes of abnormal FDG uptake in the chest have been reported, including radiation change, drug-related changes, ablation, postbiopsy and postoperative changes, lines, pacemakers, defibrillators, and lung transplants (Figs. 17 and 18).

It is common to see decreased FDG uptake in bone marrow secondary to external beam radiation to the thorax, which may persist for years following therapy (see Fig. 5); this is likely the result of radiation-induced functional suppression of the marrow. Radiation treatment can also be the cause of tissue inflammation with its associated increased FDG uptake. In rat models, it has been shown that there is an increase in tracer uptake in the lungs as early as 1 day after irradiation.[43] Investigators have described a linear relationship between the radiation dose and the uptake of FDG in patients with radiation pneumonitis several months after treatment.[44] In areas where CT shows patchy consolidation, FDG uptake in radiation pneumonitis can be moderate, and in other cases intense, usually following a well-demarcated linear boundary. Postradiation pericarditis or myocarditis may have an early or late onset. FDG uptake attributable to radiation myocarditis is usually discernible by the patient's history and the lack of normal coronary distribution. It should also correlate with the patient's radiation therapy planning field. Radiation-induced pericarditis has a diffuse pattern of FDG uptake, whereas radiation-induced esophagitis is typically associated with a linear increased pattern of tracer uptake along the esophageal wall (see Fig. 15).[18,45]

Several drugs have been shown to cause altered cardiac biodistribution of FDG, such as bezafibrate, benzodiazepines, and metformin.[18] Uptake of brown fat can be stimulated with the use of nicotine and ephedrine, and reduced with propranolol.[7] Marrow-stimulating agents, such as granulocyte colony-stimulating factor, and chemotherapeutic agents can cause diffusely increased marrow tracer uptake that can remain above baseline for up to 4 weeks after treatment (see Fig. 4).[46,47]

Radiofrequency ablation is one treatment option for patients with unresectable lung neoplasms. It is recommended that follow-up PET/CT should be performed approximately 3 months after ablation.[48] The pattern of FDG uptake at sites of

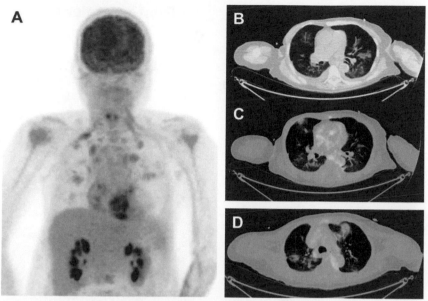

Fig. 17. (*A*) FDG-PET/CT MIP of the chest shows bilateral, mild to moderate tracer uptake in the lungs. Patchy bilateral airspace disease is seen on CT and FDG-PET/CT fusion images (*B–D*) with associated increased tracer uptake in this patient treated with chemotherapy and developed clinical findings of drug induced pneumonitis. The airspace disease and tracer uptake resolved on subsequent exams after changing the therapeutic regimen.

ablation is often more useful than its intensity during follow-up of lung lesions treated with radiofrequency ablation.[48] A diffuse, peripheral, and homogeneous pattern of uptake at the ablation site is more often associated with an inflammatory response (**Fig. 19**A, C), in contrast to the heterogeneous and focal uptake seen with lack of full response to therapy or with subsequent tumor recurrence (see **Fig. 19**B, D). Associated inflammatory uptake of FDG in the mediastinal lymph nodes has also been reported following ablation.[48]

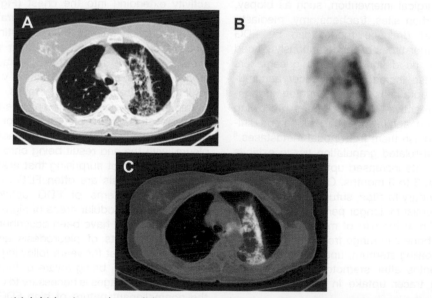

Fig. 18. Interstitial thickening and consolidative airspace disease is seen in the medial aspect of the left lung in a linear pattern on the transaxial CT image of the chest (*A*). FDG-PET and FDG-PET/CT fusion images (*B*, *C*, respectively) show moderate to high tracer uptake in the areas of airspace disease in this patient who had been previously treated with external beam radiation. This well-demarcated linear boundary and geographic pattern of tracer distribution is typical of radiation pneumonitis.

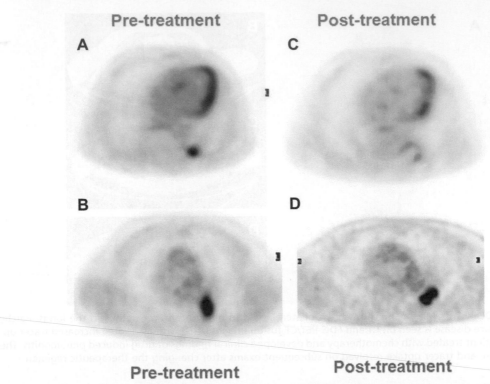

Pre-treatment   Post-treatment

Fig. 19. Transaxial FDG-PET images before (*A*, *B*) and 2 months after radiofrequency ablation (*C*, *D*) of lung cancer in 2 different patients. (*C*) Diffuse, peripheral, and homogeneous pattern of uptake surrounding a photopenic center in the treated left lung lesion, compatible with a good treatment response to ablation. (*D*) Posttreatment image showing lack of response to ablation characterized by persistent and intense focal uptake, consistent with residual malignancy.

Sites of surgical intervention, such as biopsy, catheter-insertion sites, tracheostomy, mediastinoscopy, and drainage tubes, can be FDG avid.[8,49,50] Other types of percutaneously placed devices such as defibrillators and pacemakers can also cause increased radiotracer accumulation. FDG uptake is not uncommon in nonmalignant (reactive) lymph nodes following instrumentation, and in some cases it can be difficult to distinguish them from nodal metastases.[8] Posttreatment-related granulation tissue exhibits mild to moderate increased uptake that tends to resolve within 3 to 6 months. On the other hand, uptake secondary to clips, sutures, and tracheotomies can persist for longer periods.

FDG uptake at the site of median sternotomy and healing bone can range from mild to moderate. In the healing sternum, uptake may be seen up to 6 months after sternotomy and typically has uniform tracer uptake in the craniocaudal direction.[8]

When mediastinoscopy is performed before PET/CT imaging in a patient with lung cancer, the biopsy-tract changes are easily recognized by their typical linear, moderate to intense FDG activity extending into the chest (**Fig. 20**). This pattern is consistent with the postoperative inflammatory reaction caused by mediastinoscopy. If reactive changes have occurred in unsampled lymph nodes, the resulting low to moderate increase in nodal uptake can make it very difficult to distinguish from nodal metastases.

Talc pleurodesis is commonly performed for palliation of recurrent pleural effusions. Talc induces an intense inflammatory reaction in the pleura, with the end result being chronic fibrosis. Therefore, it is not surprising that areas affected by talc pleurodesis are often FDG avid.[51] Focal and diffuse patterns of FDG uptake in both plaque-like and nodular areas of high-attenuation pleural thickening have been described.[51] The inflammatory effects of pleurodesis and its FDG avidity may persist for years following the procedure.[51] Therefore, being aware of these patterns in CT and PET images is necessary to characterize the nonmalignant nature of high FDG uptake in pleurodesis-induced granulomatous reactions.

In lung transplant recipients, FDG-PET can be used to help differentiate between rejection and infection, as the latter is characterized by an

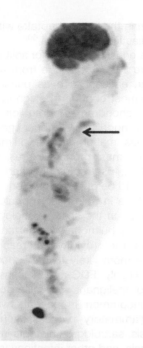

Fig. 20. Right lateral FDG-PET MIP image shows a moderately to intense linear pattern of FDG activity extending from the level of the suprasternal notch into the chest toward FDG-avid mediastinal adenopathy (*arrow*). This linear uptake is consistent with mediastinoscopy-induced inflammatory tract changes extending from the site of scope insertion.

FDG-avid neutrophilic response.[52] Based on this, it has been proposed that PET should be used to reduce the number of biopsies required after lung transplantation.[52] On the other hand, there is minimal variation in the intensity of tracer uptake in patients with rejection of a lung transplant.[53]

Sarcoidosis

Sarcoidosis is a multisystem disease, which can involve the lung parenchyma, lymph nodes, and even the heart. Sarcoidosis causes noncaseating granulomas, and its etiology is unknown. Intensity of FDG uptake has been suggested to be related to the activity of the disease. The FDG-PET lung sarcoid pattern is usually consistent with intense and diffuse FDG uptake in areas of peribronchovascular nodularity, coupled with focal uptake in bilateral lymphadenopathy and moderate to high FDG avidity in the areas of subpleural nodularity (**Fig. 21**). Differentiating noninfectious granulomatous disease caused by sarcoidosis from infectious granulomatous disease due to tuberculosis and from lymphoma is necessary to guide proper clinical management. Therefore, considering that FDG-PET cannot reliably distinguish between malignancy (eg, lymphangitic carcinomatosis) and sarcoidosis or tuberculosis, it should only be used after a diagnosis has been made.[50] Cardiac sarcoidosis can also be evaluated with PET. Most protocols involve perfusion imaging coupled

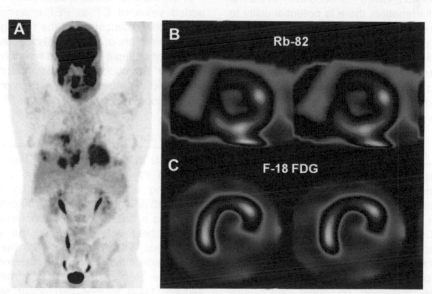

Fig. 21. (*A*) FDG-PET/CT MIP image shows patchy diffuse tracer uptake in the lung parenchyma bilaterally and heterogeneous myocardial FDG accumulation in a patient being evaluated for sarcoidosis. (*B*) ^{82}Rb myocardial perfusion short-axis images demonstrate a perfusion defect in the mid-anteroseptal and anterior left ventricular walls. (*C*) Corresponding FDG images show increased tracer uptake in the hypoperfused myocardial segments. This mismatch between myocardial perfusion and metabolism observed after proper dietary preparation (as described in the text) is both sensitive and specific for myocardial sarcoidosis. ([*B*] *Courtesy of* Hicham Skali, MD, Brigham and Women's Hospital, Boston, MA.)

with FDG-PET of the heart, preceded by specific patient preparation to control for variable glucose or use of free fatty acids by the myocardium (eg, prolonged fasting, heparin use, and high-fat low-carbohydrate diets).[54] Although cardiac FDG uptake patterns can be variable in sarcoidosis, the prevalence of focal and focal on diffuse patterns of uptake in the myocardium was reported to be more common in patients with sarcoidosis.[54] A meta-analysis evaluating the accuracy of FDG-PET for the diagnosis of cardiac sarcoidosis revealed sensitivity of 89% and specificity of 78%, underscoring the potential of FDG-PET to diagnose, direct patient management, and monitor response to therapy in patients with cardiac sarcoidosis.[55]

Cystic Fibrosis

Cystic fibrosis is an autosomal recessive disease, most commonly caused by a deletion in the gene cystic fibrosis transmembrane conductance regulator (CFTR) that causes deregulation of the transport of salt and chloride across epithelial membranes.[56] Patients have thick and viscous mucus secretions, which are difficult to clear from the airways and can result in chronic infections.[56] FDG-PET has been shown to be a useful tool to evaluate inflammatory changes in the affected patient population, with good correlation with lung function. Given the sensitivity of PET in detecting inflammation, there is potential utility to evaluate the effectiveness of therapeutic agents.[57] In fact, the change in SUV_{max} between baseline and posttreatment PET in areas of focal uptake in the affected lung zones was shown to have a negative and significant correlation with the forced expiratory volume in 1 second, and a positive correlation with cystic fibrosis CT scores.[57]

Pulmonary Nodules

By definition, a solitary pulmonary nodule is an oval or round parenchymal opacity of less than 3 cm in diameter, surrounded by normal lung in the absence of adenopathy, atelectasis, or a lung infection. FDG-PET was initially approved for the characterization of solitary pulmonary nodules and the initial staging of lung cancers in the late 1990s.[58] More than 150,000 solitary pulmonary nodules are diagnosed on chest radiography each year.[59] The benefit of evaluating solitary pulmonary nodules with PET/CT is its higher but less than perfect specificity, ranging from 77% to 90%, compared with 58% for contrast-enhanced CT.[60] The images can be analyzed semiquantitatively by calculating the lesions' SUV, and/or visually by comparing the lesions' uptake with the activity in the mediastinal blood pool.[60]

The differential diagnoses for solitary pulmonary nodules are vast, and range from malignancy to rare benign entities such as pulmonary hamartoma. The most common benign causes are hamartomas, chondromas, granulomas, infection, rheumatoid nodules, Wegener granulomatosis, arteriovenous malformations, pulmonary infarctions, hematomas, bronchial atresias, pulmonary sequestration, pseudotumors, and artifacts that may appear to be of pulmonary origin.[61]

FDG uptake in pulmonary nodules is variable, and depends on the specific etiology. Benign lesions such as pulmonary hamartoma are classically low in tracer avidity, whereas inflammatory causes are more likely to have increased tracer uptake.[62] Highly FDG-avid lesions are usually considered malignant, so false-positive results are not uncommon in patients with infectious and/or inflammatory processes such as active tuberculosis, sarcoidosis, histoplasmosis, coccidioidomycosis, and other infections (see **Fig. 16**).[60] Therefore, FDG-positive nodules always require further histologic assessment. Last but not least, during the acute and subacute phases of pulmonary emboli and infarcts, FDG uptake can be in the mild to moderate range, and therefore must be carefully distinguished from malignancy (**Fig. 22**).

In the case of multiple pulmonary nodules, the added value of CT to PET imaging allows for further characterization of the findings based on the distribution of the nodules. A tree-and-bud pattern of multiple nodules is typically associated with an infectious or inflammatory process, compared with the random pattern of distribution of centrilobular pulmonary nodules.[62]

Chest Trauma

Trauma is the leading cause of death in patients between the age of 1 and 55 years, and is increasing worldwide, accounting for approximately 25% of trauma-related deaths.[63,64] Chest trauma is a broad term that encompasses injury to the chest wall, the lungs, the airways, the esophagus, vascular structures, the heart, and other mediastinal organs.[63] Contusions and fractures are among the most common chest-wall injuries. Lung injuries can occur secondary to contusions, lacerations, pneumothorax, and hemothorax. Airway injury can result in tracheobronchial tear, while transection and dissection are common vascular injuries resulting from trauma. The heart can be contused, have decreased function secondary to tamponade, or even suffer

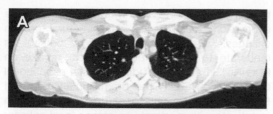

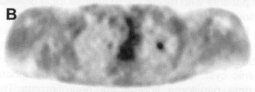

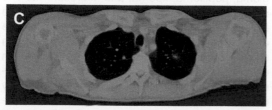

Fig. 22. (A) Transaxial noncontrast enhanced CT, (B) FDG-PET, and (C) FDG-PET/CT fusion images show a focal region of FDG uptake in the left upper lung lobe. This patient underwent subsequent CT with contrast that showed a corresponding pulmonary embolus. Variable tracer uptake can be seen in cases such as this, and localization to the pulmonary artery on fusion images is important in differentiating an FDG-avid embolus from a metabolically active pulmonary nodule.

myocardial arrest. Acute fractures and soft-tissue injuries such as contusions are FDG avid. Fortunately, FDG uptake attributable to trauma of the soft tissues of the chest wall is typically lower than in malignancy.[65] Increased FDG avidity has also been reported in patients with posttraumatic

lung contusion.[42] On the other hand, decreased FDG myocardial metabolism in an area of decreased perfusion has been described in patients diagnosed with posttraumatic myocardial contusion.[66]

Myocardium and Great Vessels

The use of FDG-PET for the evaluation of myocardial viability is a well-established tool, and probably one of the most sensitive noninvasive techniques to predict left ventricular function after coronary revascularization.[67,68,69,70] Typically patients undergoing PET imaging are loaded with oral glucose and then may receive insulin following institutional protocol. The main goal is to augment FDG uptake in the suspected hibernating myocardium to differentiate it from nonmetabolically active scar. When myocardial FDG-PET is coupled with perfusion imaging, a metabolism-perfusion mismatch (FDG uptake in hypoperfused myocardium) is considered the hallmark of myocardial viability.

Increased FDG uptake in the atrium has been associated with lipomatous hypertrophy of the interatrial septum and atrial fibrillation (**Fig. 23**). Lipomatous hypertrophy of the interatrial septum is associated with a fatty mass on CT.[18] Thrombus can be found in the atria of patients with atrial fibrillation as well as in a thrombosed vascular aneurysm. Thrombus formation results from platelet activation and adhesion of white blood cells, which are known to accumulate FDG.[71]

Tracer uptake in the aorta has been described in atherosclerotic-related disease. Atherosclerotic vessels have oxidized low-density lipoproteins accumulating in the endothelium, with subsequent endothelial dysfunction. This dysfunction causes

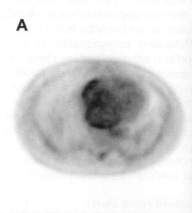

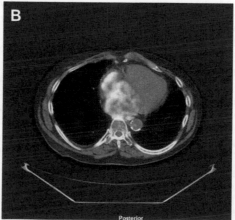

Fig. 23. (A) Transaxial FDG-PET and (B) corresponding FDG-PET/CT fusion images through the level of the heart demonstrate increased tracer uptake in the right and left atria in a patient with known atrial fibrillation.

inflammatory cell migration and activation, with the associated increased FDG uptake.[71] It is therefore postulated that areas of active atherosclerosis in the thoracic aorta will have increased tracer accumulation. Increased tracer uptake in the coronary arteries has also been proposed as a tool to estimate the degree of inflammation in the vulnerable atherosclerotic plaque, following patient preparation with a low-carbohydrate, high-fat meal the night before and a vegetable oil drink the morning of the study.[72]

Aortitis is an inflammatory condition characterized by increased FDG uptake in the affected vessel wall. FDG-PET may play a role in the early detection of aortitis given its sensitivity, and in monitoring treatment response.[71]

Aortic dissection is a common, potentially life-threatening condition. Dissections can be acute or chronic. FDG-PET can differentiate the acuity of the dissection and help provide risk-stratification information.[73] Higher uptake correlates with an increased risk for rupture and progression.[74] Furthermore, it has been shown that acute dissections can be differentiated from their chronic and stable counterparts by quantifying the SUV ratio of aortic to blood-pool uptake.[73]

FDG-PET has been used to interrogate the degree of cellular metabolism in the setting of pulmonary hypertension.[75] Investigators showed that despite elevated right ventricular and lung parenchymal FDG uptake in patients with pulmonary artery hypertension, the pulmonary arteries have normal levels of the radiotracer. The observed elevated uptake in the right ventricle and lungs, without increased uptake in the pulmonary arteries, suggests that the process is likely secondary to the distal vasculature.[75]

Esophagitis, Barrett Esophagus, and Benign Esophageal Masses

The normal esophagus may show mild normal uptake related to smooth muscle activity.[45,76] Inflammatory conditions of the esophagus are generally FDG avid, as is seen in the case of both gastroesophageal reflux and postradiation-induced inflammation (see Fig. 15). Although infrequent, high esophageal uptake was found to correlate with the coexistence of a hiatal hernia in a study of 500 patients who underwent PET/CT and endoscopy.[77] Mild distal esophageal uptake near the gastroesophageal junction is a well-known source of false-positive and false-negative results when using PET to diagnose esophageal adenocarcinoma.[45] Barrett esophagus is considered an adaptation to chronic acid exposure from reflux esophagitis. The progression of Barrett metaplasia

to malignancy correlates with changes in gene expression, as well as with structural protein changes.[78] Barrett esophagus may present as moderate to intense focal or linear uptake on FDG-PET in an area of diffuse distal esophageal thickening on CT.[79] The premalignant nature of Barrett metaplasia calls for endoscopic correlation in patients with moderate to intense focal or linear esophageal uptake if clinically indicated.[79]

Benign esophageal masses include leiomyoma, hemangioma, granular cell tumors, congenital esophageal cyst, fibrovascular polyps, bronchogenic cyst, inflammatory fibroid polyp, lymphangioma, papilloma, lipoma, and neurofibroma. The most common is the leiomyoma, which can be FDG avid and thus can become a probable source of false-positive results.[79,80] FDG-PET has been shown to be a useful tool to differentiate benign esophageal masses from early esophageal carcinoma. The best differentiators of benign from early malignant lesions are the focality and the eccentricity of the FDG uptake in the cancerous mass.[76]

Benign Conditions Affecting the Trachea

Benign tumors of the trachea include hamartomas, papillomas, lipomas, leiomyomas, and neurogenic tumors. These tumors are rare, and account for less than 10% of airway neoplasms. The most common are hamartomas and papillomas. Although these benign lesions may have some degree of FDG avidity, it is typically less so than in malignant tumors.[81]

Tracheal diverticulum is a rare entity that may be congenital or acquired. Normally these are benign air-filled outpouchings arising from the trachea, and are not FDG avid. However, if the diverticulum is infected there may be associated increased FDG uptake.[82]

Postintubation stenosis of the trachea is caused by reactive granulation tissue following prolonged intubation, and may be mildly FDG avid.[8,83]

Relapsing polychondritis is an inflammatory condition affecting cartilage throughout the body. In active disease increased tracer accumulation can be seen in the cartilages throughout the chest, including the rib cartilages, larynx, trachea, and major bronchi. FDG uptake resolves after appropriate management.[84,85] Identification of airway involvement early in the disease course may allow for delay or prevention of cartilaginous destruction and associated complications.[85]

Elastofibroma Dorsi

Elastofibroma dorsi is a relatively common, benign, slow-growing pseudotumor located along the inferior subscapular region, deep to serratus

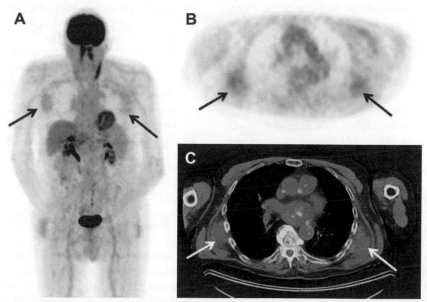

Fig. 24. (*A*) FDG-PET/CT MIP and (*B*) transaxial FDG-PET images show nearly symmetric and mild FDG uptake (*arrows*) corresponding to (*C*) poorly circumscribed soft-tissue masses in the infrascapular regions on the FDG-PET/CT fusion image (*arrows*).

anterior, and often attached to the periosteum of the ribs. These tumors are characterized by excessive fibroblast proliferation and abnormal accumulation of elastic fiber, leading to swelling, pain, and discomfort. Mild to moderate FDG uptake is frequently observed in these masses, which can become the source of false-positive findings (**Fig. 24**). Therefore, PET findings are to be correlated with those of CT. Their characteristic CT appearance is that of a poorly circumscribed soft-tissue mass, with attenuation near that of muscle, and in the typical location.[86]

Amyloidosis

Amyloidosis in the chest may affect the tracheobronchial tree, pulmonary parenchyma, pleura, or heart. The disease is characterized by the abnormal extracellular deposition of amyloid.[29] There appears to be a somewhat variable uptake of FDG in amyloidosis affecting the chest. Case reports have been published describing intense FDG avidity in nodular pulmonary and tracheobronchial tree disease.[87,88] Others have encountered negative FDG-PET findings in pulmonary and cardiac disease.[89] Further investigation is needed to elucidate the exact role of FDG-PET in this disease entity.

SUMMARY

When relying on FDG-PET/CT imaging to characterize the nature of thoracic indeterminate findings

on conventional imaging modalities, it should always be kept in mind that FDG's distribution is not merely limited to malignant lesions. Familiarity with the normal thoracic biodistribution of FDG, coupled with knowledge of the potential benign causes of increased FDG uptake in the thorax, is essential in minimizing the incidence of incorrect interpretation of FDG-PET images in daily clinical practice.

REFERENCES

1. Rohren EM, Turkington TG, Coleman RE. Clinical applications of PET in oncology. Radiology 2004; 231(2):305–32.
2. Saif MW, Tzannou I, Makrilia N, et al. Role and cost effectiveness of PET/CT in management of patients with cancer. Yale J Biol Med 2010;83(2):53–65.
3. Yang SN, Liang JA, Lin FJ, et al. Differentiating benign and malignant pulmonary lesions with FDG-PET. Anticancer Res 2001;21(6A):4153–7.
4. Alavi A, Gupta N, Alberini JL, et al. Positron emission tomography imaging in nonmalignant thoracic disorders. Semin Nucl Med 2002;32(4):293–321.
5. Kapucu LO, Meltzer CC, Townsend DW, et al. Fluorine-18-fluorodeoxyglucose uptake in pneumonia. J Nucl Med 1998;39(7):1267–9.
6. Vranjesevic D, Schiepers C, Silverman DH, et al. Relationship between ^{18}F-FDG uptake and breast density in women with normal breast tissue. J Nucl Med 2003;44:1238–42.

7. Paidisetty S, Blodgett TM. Brown fat: atypical locations and appearances encountered in PET/CT. AJR Am J Roentgenol 2009;193(2):359–66.

8. Shreve PD, Anzai Y, Wahl RL. Pitfalls in oncologic diagnosis with FDG PET imaging: physiologic and benign variants. Radiographics 1999;19(1):61–77.

9. Shammas A, Lim R, Charron M. Pediatric FDG PET/CT: physiologic uptake, normal variants, and benign conditions. Radiographics 2009;29(5):1467–86.

10. Barrington SF, Maisey MN. Skeletal muscle uptake of fluorine-18-FDG: effect of oral diazepam. J Nucl Med 1996;37(7):1127–9.

11. Yasuda S, Ide M, Takagi S, et al. Elevated F-18 FDG uptake in skeletal muscle. Clin Nucl Med 1998;23(2):111–2.

12. Nakatani K, Nakamoto Y, Togashi K. Risk factors for extensive skeletal muscle uptake in oncologic FDG-PET/CT for patients undergoing a 4-h fast. Nucl Med Commun 2012;33(6):648–55.

13. Benard F, Sterman D, Smith RJ, et al. Metabolic imaging of malignant pleural mesothelioma with fluorodeoxyglucose positron emission tomography. Chest 1998;114(3):713–22.

14. Gerbaudo VH, Julius B. Anatomo-metabolic characteristics of atelectasis in F-18 FDG-PET/CT imaging. Eur J Radiol 2007;64(3):401–5.

15. Nakahara T, Fujii H, Ide M, et al. FDG uptake in the morphologically normal thymus: comparison of FDG positron emission tomography and CT. Br J Radiol 2001;74(885):821–4.

16. Ferdinand B, Gupta P, Kramer EL. Spectrum of thymic uptake at ^{18}F-FDG PET. Radiographics 2004;24(6):1611–6.

17. Sasaki M, Kuwabara Y, Ichiya Y, et al. Differential diagnosis of thymic tumors using a combination of ^{11}C-methionine PET and FDG PET. J Nucl Med 1999;40(10):1595–601.

18. Maurer AH, Burshteyn M, Adler LP, et al. How to differentiate benign versus malignant cardiac and paracardiac ^{18}F FDG uptake at oncologic PET/CT. Radiographics 2011;31(5):1287–305.

19. Brigid GA, Flanagan FL, Dehdashti F. Whole-body positron emission tomography: normal variations, pitfalls, and technical considerations. AJR Am J Roentgenol 1997;169:1675–80.

20. Kwan A, Seltzer M, Czernin J, et al. Characterization of hilar lymph node by ^{18}F-fluoro-2-deoxyglucose positron emission tomography in healthy subjects. Anticancer Res 2001;21(1B):701–6.

21. Karam M, Roberts-Klein S, Shet N, et al. Bilateral hilar foci on ^{18}F-FDG PET scan in patients without lung cancer: variables associated with benign and malignant etiology. J Nucl Med 2008;49(9):1429–36.

22. Jeung MY, Gangi A, Gasser B, et al. Imaging of chest wall disorders. Radiographics 1999;19(3):617–37.

23. Love C, Tomas MB, Tronco GG, et al. FDG PET of infection and inflammation. Radiographics 2005;25(5):1357–68.

24. Osinowo O, Adebo OA, Okbanjo AO. Osteomyelitis of the ribs in Ibadan. Thorax 1986;41:58–60.

25. Mader JT, Shirtliff M, Calhoun JH. The host and the skeletal infection: classification and pathogenesis of acute bacterial bone and joint sepsis. Baillieres Best Pract Res Clin Rheumatol 1999;13(1):1–20.

26. Termaat MF, Raijmakers PG, Scholten HJ, et al. The accuracy of diagnostic imaging for the assessment of chronic osteomyelitis: a systematic review and meta-analysis. J Bone Joint Surg Am 2005;87(11):2464–71.

27. Ajdinovic B, Jaukovic L, Antoniou D. Five benign myoskeletal diseases in paediatrics and the role of nuclear medicine. Do they differ from those in adults? Hell J Nucl Med 2013;16(1):2–8.

28. Marik PE. Aspiration pneumonitis and aspiration pneumonia. N Engl J Med 2001;344(9):665–71.

29. Asad S, Aquino SL, Piyavisetpat N, et al. False-positive FDG positron emission tomography uptake in nonmalignant chest abnormalities. AJR Am J Roentgenol 2004;182(4):983–9.

30. Athanassiadi KA. Infections of the mediastinum. Thorac Surg Clin 2009;19(1):37–45.

31. Yen RF, Chen YC, Wu YW, et al. Using 18-fluoro-2-deoxyglucose positron emission tomography in detecting infectious endocarditis/endoarteritis: a preliminary report. Acad Radiol 2004;11(3):316–21.

32. Ha JW, Lee JD, Ko YG, et al. Images in cardiovascular medicine. Assessment of pericardial inflammation in a patient with tuberculous effusive constrictive pericarditis with ^{18}F-2-deoxyglucose positron emission tomography. Circulation 2006;113(1):e4–5.

33. Takano H, Nakagawa K, Ishio N, et al. Active myocarditis in a patient with chronic active Epstein-Barr virus infection. Int J Cardiol 2008;130(1):e11–3.

34. Raghu G, Brown KK. Interstitial lung disease: clinical evaluation and keys to an accurate diagnosis. Clin Chest Med 2004;25:409–19.

35. Groves AM, Win T, Screaton NJ, et al. Idiopathic pulmonary fibrosis and diffuse parenchymal lung disease: implications from initial experience with ^{18}F-FDG PET/CT. J Nucl Med 2009;50(4):538–45.

36. Capobianco J, Grimberg A, Thompson BM, et al. Thoracic manifestations of collagen vascular diseases. Radiographics 2012;32(1):33–50.

37. Brown KK. Pulmonary vasculitis. Proc Am Thorac Soc 2006;3(1):48–57.

38. Reichert M, Bensadoun ES. PET imaging in patients with coal workers pneumoconiosis and suspected malignancy. J Thorac Oncol 2009;4:649–51.

39. Chung SY, Lee JH, Kim TH, et al. ^{18}F-FDG PET imaging of progressive massive fibrosis. Ann Nucl Med 2010;24:21–7.

40. Ozkan M, Ayan A, Arik D, et al. FDG PET findings in a case with acute pulmonary silicosis. Ann Nucl Med 2009;23:883–6.

41. Jacene HA, Cohade C, Wahl RL. F-18 FDG PET/CT in acute respiratory distress syndrome: a case report. Clin Nucl Med 2004;29(12):786–8.

42. Rodrigues RS, Miller PR, Bozza FA, et al. FDG-PET in patients at risk for acute respiratory distress syndrome: a preliminary report. Intensive Care Med 2008;34(12):2273–8.

43. Kesner AL, Lau VK, Speiser M, et al. Time-course of effects of external beam radiation on [18F]FDG uptake in healthy tissue and bone marrow. J Appl Clin Med Phys 2008;9(3):2747.

44. McCurdy MR, Castillo R, Martinez J, et al. [18F]-FDG uptake dose-response correlates with radiation pneumonitis in lung cancer patients. Radiother Oncol 2012;104(1):52–7.

45. Kostakoglu L, Agress H Jr, Goldsmith SJ. Clinical role of FDG PET in evaluation of cancer patients. Radiographics 2003;23(2):315–40.

46. Baba S, Tatsumi M, Ishimori T, et al. Effect of nicotine and ephedrine on the accumulation of ^{18}F-FDG in brown adipose tissue. J Nucl Med 2007;48(6):981–6.

47. Cohade C. Altered biodistribution on FDG-PET with emphasis on brown fat and insulin effect. Semin Nucl Med 2010;40(4):283–93.

48. Deandreis D, Leboulleux S, Dromain C, et al. Role of FDG PET/CT and chest CT in the follow-up of lung lesions treated with radiofrequency ablation. Radiology 2011;258(1):270–6.

49. Carter KR, Kotlyarov E. Common causes of false positive F18 FDG PET/CT scans in oncology. Braz Arch Biol Technol 2007;50:29–35.

50. El-Haddad G, Zhuang H, Gupta N, et al. Evolving role of positron emission tomography in the management of patients with inflammatory and other benign disorders. Semin Nucl Med 2004;34(4):313–29.

51. Kwek BH, Aquino SL, Fischman AJ. Fluorodeoxyglucose positron emission tomography and CT after talc pleurodesis. Chest 2004;125:2356.

52. Jones HA, Donovan T, Goddard MJ, et al. Use of [18]FDG-PET to discriminate between infection and rejection in lung transplant recipients. Transplantation 2004;77(9):1462–4.

53. de Prost N, Tucci MR, Melo MF. Assessment of lung inflammation with ^{18}F-FDG PET during acute lung injury. AJR Am J Roentgenol 2010;195(2):292–300.

54. Okumura W, Iwasaki T, Toyama T, et al. Usefulness of fasting ^{18}F-FDG PET in identification of cardiac sarcoidosis. J Nucl Med 2004;45(12):1989–98.

55. Youssef G, Leung E, Mylonas I, et al. The use of ^{18}F-FDG PET in the diagnosis of cardiac sarcoidosis: a systematic review and metaanalysis including the Ontario experience. J Nucl Med 2012;53(2):241–8.

56. Torpy JM, Lynm C, Glass RM. JAMA patient page. Cystic fibrosis. JAMA 2009;302(10):1130.

57. Amin R, Charron M, Grinblat L, et al. Cystic fibrosis: detecting changes in airway inflammation with FDG PET/CT. Radiology 2012;264(3):868–75.

58. National coverage determination (NCD) for positron emission tomography (PET) scans (220.6). 2009. Available at: http://www.cms.gov/medicare-coverage-database/details/ncd-details.aspx?NCDId=211&ncdver=4&NCAId=92&ver=19&NcaName=Positron+Emission+Tomography+&bc=BEAAAAAAIAAA&. Accessed February 21, 2013.

59. Ost D, Fein AM, Feinsilver SH. Clinical practice: the solitary pulmonary nodule. N Engl J Med 2003;348:2535–42.

60. Christensen JA, Nathan MA, Mullan BP, et al. Characterization of the solitary pulmonary nodule: ^{18}F-FDG PET versus nodule-enhancement CT. AJR Am J Roentgenol 2006;187(5):1361–7.

61. Erasmus JJ, Connolly JE, McAdams HP, et al. Solitary pulmonary nodules: part I. Morphologic evaluation for differentiation of benign and malignant lesions. Radiographics 2000;20(1):43–58.

62. Bunyaviroch T, Coleman RE. PET evaluation of lung cancer. J Nucl Med 2006;47(3):451–69.

63. Centers for Disease Control and Prevention. Accidents/unintentional injuries. CDC Web site. Available at: http://www.cdc.gov/nchs/FASTATS/acc-inj.htm. Accessed February 24, 2013.

64. Mattox KL, Wall MJ Jr. Newer diagnostic measures and emergency management. Chest Surg Clin N Am 1997;7(2):213–26.

65. Kavanagh PV, Stevenson AW, Chen MY, et al. Nonneoplastic diseases in the chest showing increased activity on FDG PET. AJR Am J Roentgenol 2004;183(4):1133–41.

66. Pai M. Diagnosis of myocardial contusion after blunt chest trauma using ^{18}F-FDG positron emission tomography. Br J Radiol 2006;79(939):264–5.

67. Soussan M, Brillet PY, Nunes H, et al. Clinical value of a high-fat and low-carbohydrate diet before FDG-PET/CT for evaluation of patients with suspected cardiac sarcoidosis. J Nucl Cardiol 2013;20(1):120–7.

68. Matthews R, Bench T, Meng H, et al. Diagnosis and monitoring of cardiac sarcoidosis with delayed-enhanced MRI and ^{18}F-FDG PET-CT. J Nucl Cardiol 2012;19(4):807–10.

69. Schinkel AF, Bax JJ, Poldermans D, et al. Hibernating myocardium: diagnosis and patient outcomes. Curr Probl Cardiol 2007;32(7):375–410.

70. Vitale GD, deKemp RA, Ruddy TD, et al. Myo-cardial glucose utilization and optimization of (18) F-FDG PET imaging in patients with non-insulin-dependent diabetes mellitus, coronary artery disease, and left ventricular dysfunction. J Nucl Med 2001;42(12):1730–6.

71. Hayashida T, Sueyoshi E, Sakamoto I, et al. PET features of aortic diseases. AJR Am J Roentgenol 2010;195(1):229–33.

72. Wykrzykowska J, Lehman S, Williams G, et al. Imaging of inflamed and vulnerable plaque in coronary arteries with ^{18}F-FDG PET/CT in patients with suppression of myocardial uptake using a low-carbohydrate, high-fat preparation. J Nucl Med 2009;50(4):563–8.

73. Reeps C, Pelisek J, Bundschuh RA, et al. Imaging of acute and chronic aortic dissection by ^{18}F-FDG PET/CT. J Nucl Med 2010;51(5):686–91.

74. Kato K, Nishio A, Kato N, et al. Uptake of ^{18}F-FDG in acute aortic dissection: a determinant of unfavorable outcome. J Nucl Med 2010;51(5):674–81.

75. Hagan G, Southwood M, Treacy C, et al. (18)FDG PET imaging can quantify increased cellular metabolism in pulmonary arterial hypertension: a proof-of-principle study. Pulm Circ 2011;1(4):448–55.

76. Roedl JB, Colen RR, King K, et al. Visual PET/CT scoring for nonspecific ^{18}F-FDG uptake in the differentiation of early malignant and benign esophageal lesions. AJR Am J Roentgenol 2008;191(2):515–21.

77. Takechi M, Yasuda S, Chino O, et al. Physiologic FDG uptake in the esophagus. J Nucl Med 2008;49(Suppl 1):260P.

78. Conteduca V, Sansonno D, Ingravallo G, et al. Barrett's esophagus and esophageal cancer: an overview. Int J Oncol 2012;41(2):414–24.

79. Kamel EM, Thumshirn M, Truninger K, et al. Significance of incidental ^{18}FDG accumulations in the gastrointestinal tract in PET/CT: correlation with endoscopic and histopathologic results. J Nucl Med 2004;45(11):1804–10.

80. Meirelles GS, Ravizzini G, Yeung HW, et al. Esophageal leiomyoma: a rare cause of false-positive FDG scans. Clin Nucl Med 2006;31:342–4.

81. Park CM, Goo JM, Lee HJ, et al. Tumors in the tracheobronchial tree: CT and FDG PET features. Radiographics 2009;29(1):55–71.

82. Charest M, Sirois C, Cartier Y, et al. Infected tracheal diverticulum mimicking an aggressive mediastinal lesion on FDG PET/CT: an interesting case with review of the literature. Br J Radiol 2012;85(1009):e17–21.

83. De S, De S. Post intubation tracheal stenosis. Indian J Crit Care Med 2008;12(4):194–7.

84. Sato M, Hiyama T, Abe T, et al. F-18 FDG PET/CT in relapsing polychondritis. Ann Nucl Med 2010;24(9):687–90.

85. De Geeter F, Vandecasteele SJ. Fluorodeoxyglucose PET in relapsing polychondritis. N Engl J Med 2008;358(5):536–7.

86. Pierce JC 3rd, Henderson R. Hypermetabolism of elastofibroma dorsi on PET-CT. AJR Am J Roentgenol 2004;183(1):35–7.

87. Umeda Y, Demura Y, Takeda N, et al. FDG-PET findings of nodular pulmonary amyloidosis with a long-term observation. Nihon Kokyuki Gakkai Zasshi 2007;45(5):424–9 [in Japanese].

88. Seo JH, Lee SW, Ahn BC, et al. Pulmonary amyloidosis mimicking multiple metastatic lesions on F-18 FDG PET/CT. Lung Cancer 2010;67(3):376–9.

89. Mekinian A, Jaccard A, Soussan M, et al. Centre de Référence des Amyloses immunoglobulinémiques et autres maladies liées aux dépôts des immunoglobulines monoclonales. ^{18}F-FDG PET/CT in patients with amyloid light-chain amyloidosis: case-series and literature review. Amyloid 2012;19(2):94–8.

Abdomen
Normal Variations and Benign Conditions Resulting in Uptake on FDG-PET/CT

Katherine Zukotynski, MD[a,b], Chun K. Kim, MD[b,*]

KEYWORDS

- Normal variations • Benign findings • Abdomen • ^{18}F-Fluorodeoxyglucose PET/computed tomography • Imaging

KEY POINTS

- ^{18}F-Fluorodeoxyglucose positron emission tomography/computed tomography (FDG-PET/CT) plays an important role in the evaluation of oncology patients; to interpret images reliably, it is important to be familiar with normal variations and patterns of physiologic FDG uptake.
- Physiologic activity or uptake resulting from benign conditions of the genitourinary or gastrointestinal tracts is common and can obscure primary malignancy, lymphoma, or metastases.
- Artifacts from PET and CT image misregistration, motion, or metallic implants can obscure pathologic features.
- Brown adipose tissue, skeletal muscle activity, and medication can give rise to FDG uptake, and underlines the importance of knowing the clinical history at the time of FDG-PET/CT interpretation.

INTRODUCTION

^{18}F-Fluorodeoxyglucose positron emission tomography/computed tomography (FDG-PET/CT) is becoming increasingly ubiquitous as a tool for staging and follow-up of patients with carcinoma. Physiologic activity in the gastrointestinal (GI) and genitourinary (GU) tracts is common and, although often a benign pattern of activity is seen, this can limit the sensitivity of the study for the detection of FDG-avid disease. Furthermore, because abnormalities may be either FDG-avid or non–FDG-avid, close attention to both the CT and PET portions of the study must be given to ensure accurate interpretation. Several benign conditions such as metabolically active brown adipose tissue, skeletal muscle activity, medications, and inflammatory or infectious processes can present confounding factors in the evaluation of oncologic FDG-PET/CT,

and underline the need for attention to the medical history. In addition, artifacts may be encountered, often resulting from misregistration of PET and CT images arising from patient motion during image acquisition or related to metal implants. Close attention to both the CT and PET images of the PET/CT study and review of prior imaging can often help in determining whether the abnormality is related to artifact. Rarely, delayed images or short-interval follow-up is needed for further characterization.

This article presents a brief review of normal variations in physiologic FDG uptake in the abdomen, and findings commonly seen with benign processes such as inflammation. Radiotracer activity related to metabolically active brown adipose tissue, muscle activity, and medication is mentioned, and potential remedies to mitigate these effects

[a] Department of Medical Imaging, Sunnybrook Health Sciences Centre, 2075 Bayview Avenue, University of Toronto, Toronto, Ontario M4N 3M5, Canada; [b] Division of Nuclear Medicine and Molecular Imaging, Department of Radiology, Brigham and Women's Hospital, Harvard Medical School, 75 Francis Street, Boston, MA 02115, USA
* Corresponding author. Division of Nuclear Medicine and Molecular Imaging, Department of Radiology, Brigham and Women's Hospital, 75 Francis Street, Boston, MA 02115, USA
E-mail address: ckkim@bwh.harvard.edu

PET Clin 9 (2014) 169–183
http://dx.doi.org/10.1016/j.cpet.2013.10.008
1556-8598/14/$ – see front matter © 2014 Elsevier Inc. All rights reserved.

discussed. The article concludes with a short review of artifacts that can be encountered in abdominal imaging with FDG-PET/CT.

VARIATIONS IN PHYSIOLOGIC FDG ACTIVITY IN THE ABDOMEN ON FDG-PET/CT

Physiologic FDG activity in the abdominal organs is variable. Typically there is mild diffuse FDG activity in the blood pool, bone marrow, and abdominal organs, with slightly more intense activity in the liver than in the remaining solid organs or bone marrow. Physiologic activity in the GI and GU tracts is commonly seen; this can be intense, moderate, mild, focal, segmental, and/or diffuse, and can significantly limit the sensitivity of the study for the detection of FDG-avid disease. The biological determinants of variable physiologic FDG activity in the abdomen are unknown, but might be due to several factors. In the GI and GU tract, such factors may include peristalsis during the uptake period, anatomic variations resulting in slight differences of radiotracer flow (ie, in the ureter), bacterial flora (ie, in the colon) and/or debris (ie, stool).

GI Tract

Variations in GI-tract FDG activity are common (**Fig. 1**), often benign, and are related to lymphoid

tissue, inflammation, muscular contraction, sloughed cells, medication, attenuation correction, or motion artifact.[1,2] Physiologic activity is typically mild to moderate and diffuse, whereas focal intense activity is often related to pathologic conditions, either benign or malignant (**Fig. 2**). A recent study by Jadvar[3] of 50 patients without known or suspected colonic abnormality referred for oncologic FDG-PET/CT found that colonic FDG activity was variable but often mild and diffuse, with the rectosigmoid colon having the highest median activity, followed by the cecum, ascending colon, transverse colon, and descending colon. Although intense FDG activity in the colon may be physiologic, it can suggest colitis or diverticulitis when the activity correlates with wall thickening and inflammatory changes on CT (**Fig. 3**). Moreover, FDG-PET/CT can serve as a tool to assess the extent of inflammatory bowel disease (either Crohn's disease or ulcerative colitis) and response to therapy.[4–6] Focal FDG activity in the colon can be a normal variant; however, its presence raises concern for primary colonic abnormality, often a colonic polyp (**Fig. 4**), particularly when the focal activity is intense. In a study by Tatlidil and colleagues,[7] focal intense FDG activity in the colon had a greater than 79% probability of correlating with a histopathologic abnormality such as a colonic polyp or colonic adenocarcinoma. Several

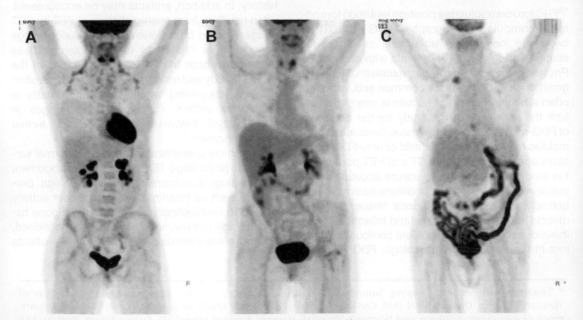

Fig. 1. Spectrum of normal variations in gastrointestinal (GI)-tract ^{18}F-fluorodeoxyglucose (FDG) uptake on PET/computed tomography (CT). (*A*) Maximum-intensity projection (MIP) image from FDG-PET/CT in an 18-year-old woman with lymphoma after therapy shows virtually absent FDG uptake in the GI tract. (*B*) MIP image from FDG-PET/CT in a 74-year-old woman with lung cancer after therapy shows mild FDG uptake in the hepatic flexure and transverse colon. (*C*) MIP image from FDG-PET/CT in an 83-year-old woman with lung cancer at staging shows diffuse intense FDG uptake throughout the entire colon, consistent with the history of metformin.

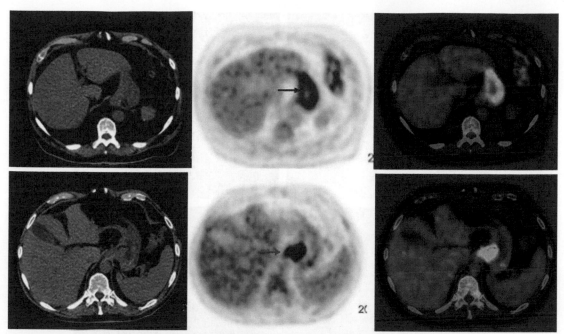

Fig. 2. Mild diffuse versus focal intense GI-tract FDG uptake on PET/CT. (*Top row*) CT, FDG-PET, and FDG-PET/CT images of a 66-year-old man with esophageal cancer show mild diffuse physiologic FDG uptake in the stomach (*blue arrow*) with no abnormality on CT. (*Bottom row*) Axial CT, FDG-PET, and fused FDG-PET/CT images of a 57-year-old man with esophageal cancer show focal intense FDG uptake in the proximal stomach (*red arrow*) correlating with soft-tissue thickening on CT at a site of known malignancy.

other studies have collectively reported incidental focal colonic uptake in 1.3% to 3.7% of FDG-PET/CT studies, and the probability that this is associated with a colonic polyp or malignant lesion is in the range of 67% to 71%.[8–10] Therefore, colonoscopy is recommended for patients referred for oncologic FDG-PET/CT found to have incidental focal activity in the colon.

In summary, mild diffuse FDG activity in the colon without a correlating CT abnormality is commonly physiologic, whereas diffuse activity with a correlating CT abnormality or intense focal activity increases the likelihood of abnormality. In

future, the possibility of correlating ex vivo FDG localization in colonic specimens with histologic findings could provide further clues to the origin of variability in colonic FDG uptake.[11]

GU Tract

Physiologic FDG activity in the GU tract without a correlating CT abnormality, including radiotracer accumulation in the renal calyces, ureters, and bladder, is commonly seen (**Fig. 5**). It is variable in appearance but often intense. This finding is benign but can obscure FDG-avid primary

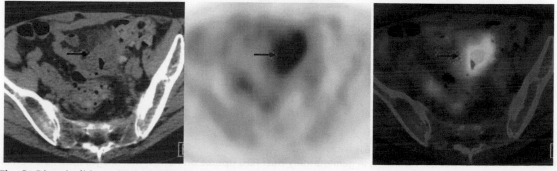

Fig. 3. Diverticulitis on FDG-PET/CT. CT, FDG-PET, and fused PET/CT images (*from left to right*) of a 52-year-old woman show intense FDG uptake in the sigmoid colon (*blue arrow*) associated with numerous diverticula and extensive inflammatory change on CT.

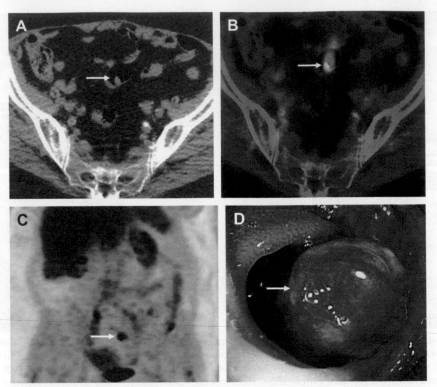

Fig. 4. Colonic polyp on FDG-PET/CT. (*A*) CT, (*B*) fused PET/CT, (*C*) MIP images, and (*D*) photo obtained at the time of colonoscopy show intense focal FDG uptake in the sigmoid colon (*arrows*) associated with a colonic polyp. (*Courtesy of* Dr K. O'Regan, BMedSci, Cork University Hospital, Cork, Ireland.)

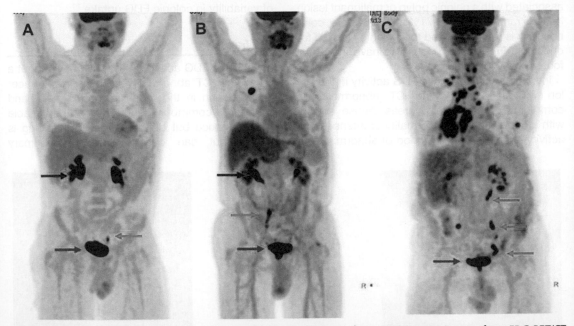

Fig. 5. Spectrum of normal variations in genitourinary tract FDG uptake on PET/CT. MIP images from FDG-PET/CT in a 35-year-old woman with lymphoma after therapy (*A*), a 75-year-old man with lung cancer at staging (*B*), and an 83-year-old man with lung cancer at staging (*C*) show the spectrum of variable physiologic FDG accumulation in the renal calyces (*blue arrows*), ureters (*green arrows*), and bladder (*red arrows*).

abnormalities of the GU tract such as transitional cell carcinoma, which are often intensely FDG-avid, or papillary urothelial carcinoma, which may have low-level activity.[12] It can also obscure FDG-avid metastatic disease or lymphoma, both of which are typically intensely FDG-avid.[13] Finally, abnormalities of the GU tract can have low-level FDG activity. As such, evaluation of the GU tract is often a blind spot for imaging specialists, and careful examination of both the PET and CT images is the key to accurate study interpretation.

Solid Organs

Physiologic FDG activity in the solid abdominal organs, including the liver, spleen, pancreas, and adrenal glands, without a correlating CT abnormality is often mild, diffuse, homogeneous, and slightly more intense in the liver than in the remaining organs (**Fig. 6**). FDG activity may appear heterogeneous depending on several factors such as the patient's body habitus and blood glucose level, and technical parameters for the study.[14,15]

Abdominal hernias are commonly seen after surgery and typically contain fat or loops of bowel (see **Fig. 6**). If herniated bowel loops are seen, it is important to look for evidence of obstruction or

inflammation. The presence of intense focal activity or a CT abnormality in the solid organs of the abdomen raises concern for pathologic status. Benign pathology can be FDG-avid, but typically photopenic or mildly FDG-avid lesions are benign whereas intensely FDG-avid lesions suggest malignant disease (**Fig. 7**). In some cases, quantitative kinetic parameters on FDG-PET/CT may suggest tumor aggressiveness.[16]

Adrenal nodules or masses are commonly identified on FDG-PET/CT. Several studies have evaluated the utility of FDG-PET/CT for distinguishing benign from malignant adrenal lesions based on intensity of FDG uptake. Yun and colleagues[17] first reported the utility of FDG-PET for evaluation of adrenal lesions seen on CT or magnetic resonance (MR) imaging in patients with known malignancies, and found that the presence of a CT abnormality such as a nodule or mass coupled with intense activity, significantly higher than liver activity, suggested malignancy. A study by Ozcan Kara and colleagues[18] of 81 patients with malignancy referred for FDG-PET/CT, including 104 adrenal lesions of which 70 were malignant and 34 were benign, reported the ratio of adrenal lesion maximum standardized uptake value (SUV) to mean liver SUV was 3.61 ± 1.77 for malignant

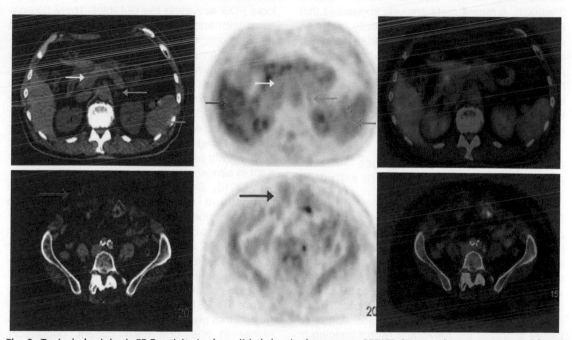

Fig. 6. Typical physiologic FDG activity in the solid abdominal organs on PET/CT. (*Top row*) CT, FDG-PET, and fused PET/CT images show physiologic mild, diffuse, homogeneous FDG uptake in the liver (*red arrow*), spleen (*green arrow*), splenule (*green arrowhead*), adrenal glands (*orange arrow*), and pancreas (*white arrow*), with slightly more intense FDG uptake in the liver compared with the other solid abdominal organs and no abnormality on CT. (*Bottom row*) CT, FDG-PET, and fused PET/CT images show physiologic GI-tract FDG uptake including loops of bowel in an anterior abdominal wall hernia (*blue arrow*). There are no CT or PET findings to suggest bowel obstruction.

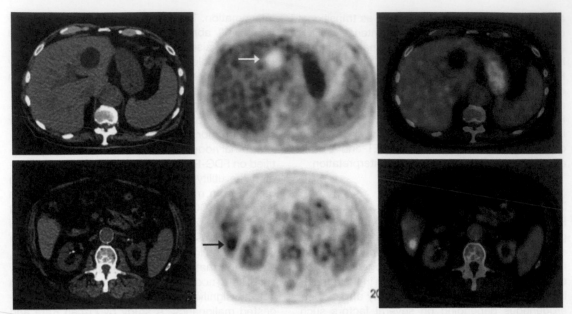

Fig. 7. Benign versus malignant hepatic disease on PET/CT. (*Top row*) CT, FDG-PET, and fused PET/CT images of a 75-year-old man with lymphoma after therapy show a photopenic hypodense well-circumscribed benign cyst (*white arrow*) in the right hepatic lobe. (*Bottom row*) CT, FDG-PET, and fused PET/CT images of a 75-year-old man with lung cancer after therapy show focal intense FDG uptake without a definite correlating CT abnormality (*black arrow*) in the right hepatic lobe at a site of known metastasis.

lesions and 1.2 ± 0.38 for benign lesions (P<.0001). A recent meta-analysis suggested that FDG-PET/CT had both high sensitivity and high specificity for differentiating benign from malignant adrenal disease.[19] Though not always the case, physiologic adrenal activity is commonly mild, homogeneous, and diffuse, benign nodules are mildly FDG-avid, and metastatic disease is intensely FDG-avid, with intense activity apparent even in very subtle lesions on CT (**Fig. 8**).

PATIENT PREPARATION TO REDUCE PHYSIOLOGIC ACTIVITY IN THE GI AND GU TRACTS

Several methods to reduce physiologic GI-tract and GU-tract FDG activity have been proposed over the years. In 1998, Miraldi and colleagues[20] suggested that an isosmotic solution be used to cleanse the colon the evening before the study, with furosemide given and a Foley catheter placed immediately before the study. Normal saline delivered to the bladder via a retrograde approach before scanning the pelvis and repeat imaging of the pelvis after voiding resulted in decreased physiologic GI-tract and GU-tract activity on PET with improved lesion detection. However, this approach is not practical, and therefore is rarely performed in the clinic. In 2006, Kamel and colleagues[21] studied the effect of forced diuresis

with parenteral hydration and voiding on physiologic FDG activity in the GU tract. Thirty-two patients with known intravesicle tumors, undefined renal lesions, or indeterminate activity in the urinary tract on an initial PET were included in the study. Following an initial PET or PET/CT, each patient received 0.5 mg furosemide per kg (maximum 40 mg) and an infusion of 500 mL normal saline intravenously over 30 minutes. Repeat PET or PET/CT of the pelvis was acquired shortly after voiding. Using this technique, intense physiologic FDG activity was eliminated from the lower urinary tract in almost all patients (97%).

In 2010, Soyka and colleagues[22] evaluated pretreatment with senna-glycoside solution to reduce physiologic intestinal activity. Sixty-five patients with abdominal malignancy referred for FDG-PET/CT were evaluated. All patients were asked to fast for 4 hours before the study. In addition, 26 patients were asked to drink 75 mL senna-glycoside solution with 2 L water by 2 PM the day before the PET/CT examination. The results suggested that physiologic bowel activity was slightly higher in the pretreated patient population, although this activity was diffuse and did not significantly impair image interpretation. Murphy and colleagues[23] studied pretreatment with 10 mL Lomotil (5 mg diphenoxylate hydrochloride/0.05 mg atropine sulfate) 30 to 60 minutes before FDG-PET/CT, and concluded that this did

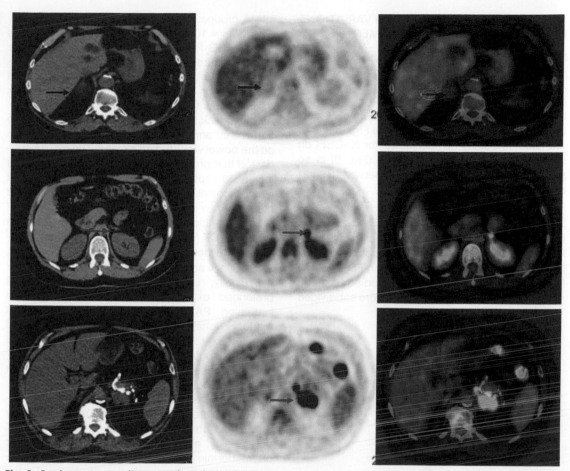

Fig. 8. Benign versus malignant adrenal gland disease on PET/CT. (*Top row*) CT, FDG-PET, and fused FDG-PET/CT images of a 79-year-old man with lung cancer at staging show a mildly FDG-avid right adrenal gland adenoma (*blue arrow*). (*Middle row*) CT, FDG-PET, and fused FDG-PET/CT images of a 47-year-old woman with lung cancer at staging show focal intense FDG uptake in a tiny left adrenal gland metastasis (*red arrow*). (*Bottom row*) CT, FDG-PET, and fused FDG-PET/CT images of a 67-year-old man with lung cancer at staging show intensely FDG-avid metastatic thickening of the left adrenal gland (*red arrow*).

not reduce physiologic FDG activity in the bowel. Jadvar and colleagues[24] evaluated colonic activity on routine FDG-PET/CT and compared this with colonic activity following the intravenous administration of atropine sulfate (to decrease peristalsis) or sincalide (to increase peristalsis). This study found no statistically significant difference between colonic activity on routine FDG-PET/CT following the administration of atropine sulfate or sincalide.

The guidelines for oncologic FDG-PET/CT available through the Society of Nuclear Medicine and Molecular Imaging do not recommend specific patient premedication or diuresis techniques to reduce physiologic GI-tract and GU-tract activity.[25] Careful attention must be paid to both the PET and CT portions of the study to ensure accurate image interpretation. Although the use of furosemide, bladder catheterization, and delayed

imaging may be helpful in certain cases, such as for the evaluation of patients with primary malignancy of the GU tract,[26,27] this is not routinely performed. In certain centers oral contrast may be used. In general, high-density barium can cause focal or diffusely increased FDG uptake, whereas low-density barium is preferred to improve anatomic delineation of bowel without introducing clinically detectable artifact.[28–30] Chun and colleagues[31] reported a case in which a PET study showed intense uptake in the rectosigmoid region suspicious for local tumor recurrence, but a repeat PET study performed after an enema a few days later showed resolution of the intense uptake in question, thus obviating surgical intervention. However, the role of the enema was unclear. Continued research into methods for reducing variations in physiologic activity and ultimately improving image interpretation are ongoing.

THE EFFECT OF MEDICATION ON VARIATIONS IN FDG ACTIVITY IN THE ABDOMEN

Medications alter cellular biology and can have a profound effect on the distribution of FDG uptake. Although a discussion of the effects of different medications on FDG uptake in the abdomen is beyond the scope of this section, the effect of metformin on activity in the GI tract (see **Fig. 1**) and of granulocyte-colony stimulating factor (G-CSF) on splenic and bone marrow activity (**Fig. 9**) is so prevalent and marked that it deserves a short discussion.

GI Tract

In a study by Massollo and colleagues[32] published in 2013, the biological response of colonic enterocytes to metformin and the effect on FDG activity in bowel seen with PET/CT was studied using 53 nondiabetic nude mice. The mice were subdivided

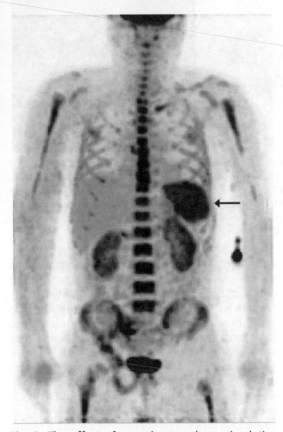

Fig. 9. The effect of granulocyte-colony stimulating factor (G-CSF) medication on FDG-PET/CT. MIP image from an FDG-PET/CT after G-CSF therapy shows diffusely increased FDG uptake in the spleen (*blue arrow*) and bone marrow. This pattern of FDG uptake is benign, but limits the sensitivity of the study for the detection of FDG-avid disease in the spleen and bone marrow.

into 4 groups: group 1 (n = 15) was untreated, group 2 (n = 10) were given metformin for 48 hours before FDG-PET/CT, group 3 (n = 10) were treated with metformin for 3 months before FDG-PET/CT, and group 4 (n = 8) were treated with metformin for 3 months and then metformin was discontinued for 48 hours before FDG-PET/CT. At the conclusion of the study, the mice were euthanized and the biological effect of metformin on the bowel was studied ex vivo. The results suggested that prolonged metformin therapy induced increased colonic wall FDG activity without altering bowel lumen FDG activity, whereas rapid changes in metformin therapy before FDG-PET/CT, either initiation of therapy for 48 hours before FDG-PET/CT (group 2) or discontinuation of therapy for 48 hours before FDG-PET/CT (group 4), did not have an appreciable effect on bowel activity. Finally, ex vivo analysis suggested that prolonged exposure to metformin resulted in increased PAMPK (phosphorylated adenosine monophosphate activated protein kinase) and reduced expression of TXNIP messenger RNA (a thioredoxin-interacting protein) in colonic enterocytes, suggesting that metformin had a direct effect on cellular biology.

Several human studies have shown that metformin typically results in intense diffuse FDG activity throughout the colon without a correlating CT abnormality, although colonic activity in patients on metformin can be variable in both intensity and pattern. In a prospective study by Gontier and colleagues[33] published in 2008, 55 patients with type 2 diabetes mellitus were divided into 2 groups, one whose treatment regimen included metformin and a second who were not exposed to metformin. The 2 groups were compared with nondiabetic control patients. The results showed a statistically significant increase in bowel FDG activity in patients exposed to metformin, with the effect being more pronounced in the large bowel than small bowel. Bybel and colleagues[34] also showed increased bowel FDG activity using a series of 77 diabetic patients, 45 of whom were being treated with metformin. The observation of increased colonic activity in patients on metformin has, in turn, led to a series of experiments designed to decrease FDG activity in bowel by discontinuing metformin before FDG-PET/CT. For example, Oh and colleagues[35] reported that discontinuing metformin for 2 days before FDG-PET/CT in 30 patients produced a significant reduction in intestinal activity. Similarly, Ozulker and colleagues[36] reported that discontinuing metformin for 3 days in 41 patients significantly reduced intestinal activity. Indeed, in the study by Oh and colleagues[35] the decrease in intestinal activity attributed to the discontinuation of metformin resulted in the detection of colorectal malignancy in 2 patients in whom this had previously been obscured. Although the literature suggests that in diabetic humans,[36] unlike nondiabetic nude mice,[32] a short period of discontinuing metformin can significantly reduce FDG activity in bowel, further research is needed to establish the biological effect of prolonged metformin use in colonic enterocytes.

Spleen and Bone Marrow

Typically, physiologic FDG activity in the abdomen includes mild diffuse activity throughout the spleen and bone marrow, at a level lower than the intensity of activity in the liver. There are several causes of diffusely increased splenic and bone marrow activity including infectious, inflammatory, and malignant etiology. Many of these processes produce accompanying CT abnormalities. Commonly encountered causes of diffusely increased splenic and bone marrow activity in oncology patients without a correlating CT abnormality, however, include elevated cytokines or medication such as G-CSF.[37–40] In a study of both animals and humans, the G-CSF medication pegfilgrastim resulted in significantly increased diffuse bone marrow and splenic activity.[41] Elevated cytokines such as interleukin (IL)-1β, IL-1 receptor antagonist, IL-4, IL-6, IL-7, and IL-13 can also cause diffusely increased splenic activity.[42]

METABOLICALLY ACTIVE BROWN ADIPOSE TISSUE, SKELETAL MUSCLE UPTAKE, AND ARTIFACTS

Physiologic variations in FDG uptake related to metabolically active brown adipose tissue and skeletal muscle activity during the uptake period may be seen throughout the abdomen. Brown adipose tissue was first described more than 450 years ago.[43] Thought to be a mechanism for nonshivering thermogenesis under sympathetic stimulation typically activated by decreased environmental temperature, brown adipose tissue may be intensely FDG-avid when metabolically active.[44,45] Although metabolically active brown adipose tissue is typically bilateral and symmetric in the neck, mediastinum, and paraspinal regions, it may be asymmetric in the abdomen, correlating with focal areas of brown adipose tissue. Common sites of metabolically active brown adipose tissue in the abdomen include the suprarenal, perinephric, and perihepatic regions (**Fig. 10**). Several

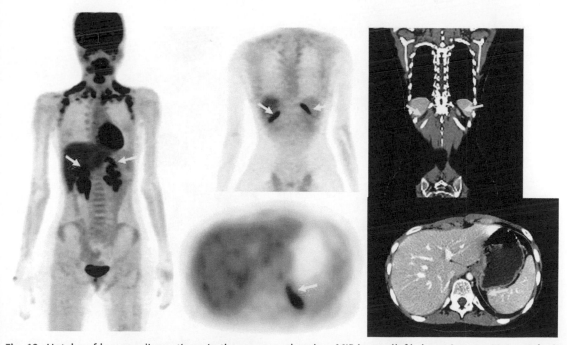

Fig. 10. Uptake of brown adipose tissue in the suprarenal region. MIP image (*left*) shows intense FDG uptake in the superclavicular and axillary regions bilaterally and the superior mediastinum, typical of uptake of brown adipose tissue. In addition, intense linear FDG uptake (*arrows*) is seen just above both kidneys. The intense linear FDG uptake seen just above both kidneys (*arrows*) on coronal (*middle above*) and transaxial (*middle below*) PET images localizes to fat on coronal (*right above*) and transaxial (*right below*) CT images, representing metabolically active brown adipose tissue in the suprarenal region.

methods have been proposed to decrease FDG activity associated with metabolically active brown adipose tissue, including patient warming through the use of ambient temperature control or warm blankets,[46–50] premedication,[51–54] or diet.[55] In general, correlation of FDG uptake with adipose tissue on CT is needed to confirm the diagnosis. Rarely, metabolically active brown adipose tissue can obscure pathologic features, and additional imaging may be needed for further characterization in these cases.

FDG uptake in skeletal muscle can also rarely obscure pathologic features. Physiologic FDG activity in skeletal muscle is typically mild, diffuse, and extends along the course of the muscle. However, if muscle activity occurs during the uptake period, linear intense FDG uptake can be seen along the course of the muscle. Moreover, increased insulin can result in diffusely increased muscle activity (**Fig. 11**). Rarely, focal activity can be seen in muscle with or without a correlating CT abnormality. Although this can reflect inflammation, often related to prior intervention, it raises concern for metastatic disease (**Fig. 12**). When focal activity is seen involving the musculoskeletal system, careful attention must be paid to the CT portion of the PET/CT study because intense

FDG activity can be seen at sites of traumatic injury, most commonly in the ribs.

Several artifacts can affect FDG-PET/CT of the abdomen. The most common artifact is attenuation correction, owing to the presence of a metal prosthesis or misregistration in CT and PET images from patient motion. Close attention to the non–attenuation-corrected images is needed to ensure apparent variations in physiologic FDG uptake on PET is due to artifact rather than to abnormality.

BENIGN CONDITIONS RESULTING IN UPTAKE ON FDG-PET/CT

FDG-avid benign infectious or inflammatory processes are often seen on oncologic PET/CT. FDG uptake may be mild to intense and, potentially, confused with a malignant process. For example, abscesses can occur throughout the abdomen and often show intense peripheral FDG uptake with central fluid-attenuation photopenia, which may be septated, unilocular, or multilocular. The presence of air bubbles or an air-fluid level suggests gas-forming organisms. Hematomas are often associated with a hemorrhagic malignancy, a coagulopathic patient, or intervention

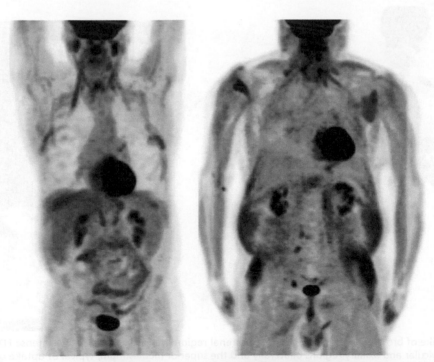

Fig. 11. Skeletal muscle uptake on FDG-PET/CT. (*Left*) MIP image from FDG-PET/CT shows FDG uptake in the accessory muscles of respiration (the patient was having difficulty breathing during the FDG uptake period). (*Right*) MIP image from FDG-PET/CT shows diffuse FDG uptake throughout the muscles in a patient with hyperinsulinemia.

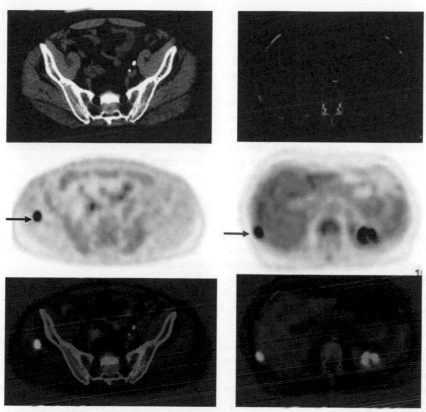

Fig. 12. Focal FDG uptake in the musculoskeletal system. (*Left*) CT, FDG-PET, and fused PET/CT images of a 68-year-old man with lung cancer at staging show focal intense FDG uptake in the right gluteal muscles without a definite correlating CT abnormality at a site of known metastasis (*blue arrow*). (*Right*) CT, FDG-PET, and fused PET/CT images of a 68-year-old man with lung cancer at staging show focal intense FDG uptake in a right rib correlating with a traumatic rib fracture on CT (*red arrow*).

(eg, biopsies, port placement), and usually consist of a central photopenic collection with mild peripheral activity. Seromas are sterile fluid collections often seen at sites of surgical intervention (eg, lymph node dissection) with a central photopenic collection and mild peripheral uptake. Ultrasonography, contrast-enhanced CT, or MR imaging may be helpful in differentiating malignancy from a hematoma or seroma. For example, on anatomic imaging hematomas and seromas are avascular, fluid-filled cavities with a thin, uniform rim of mild contrast enhancement, in contradistinction to the vascular, thick, nodular, enhancing rim, which is more commonly seen in the case of malignancy. Hematomas and seromas can be difficult to differentiate from abscesses, although faint peripheral activity suggesting little inflammation, a thin rim, and lack of air favors the diagnosis of a seroma. Sarcoidosis, tuberculosis, and fungal infections can also show a spectrum of findings on FDG-PET/CT, and typically the diagnosis can only be made based on clinical history and serial imaging follow-up confirming a waxing and waning

process or resolution over time. Retroperitoneal fibrosis is an inflammatory condition that may be idiopathic or related to prior radiation therapy, and is often associated with mildly FDG-avid lymph nodes and inflammatory change that is indistinguishable from malignancy, such as lymphoma, on a single FDG-PET/CT study.

Liver and Biliary Tract

There are numerous benign hepatobiliary lesions that can show FDG uptake. Whereas FDG uptake in benign lesions is generally lower than that in malignant lesions, such as metastatic lesions and cholangiocarcinoma, FDG uptake associated with hepatocellular carcinoma is variable, possibly related to differences in the spectrum of tumor differentiation.[56,57] Others have also reported relatively intense FDG uptake in benign liver lesions, for example, hepatic abscesses,[56] hepatic adenomas,[58] and focal nodular hyperplasia.[59] Therefore, FDG uptake alone does not seem to reliably differentiate between primary benign and primary malignant hepatic lesions. The addition of diagnostic imaging such as ultrasonography, contrast-enhanced CT, or MR imaging is often needed to characterize lesions as benign or malignant. Often clinical history is the key factor in deriving the diagnosis.

More recently, Lee and colleagues[60] assessed the value of FDG uptake in risk stratification for surgical intervention of gallbladder polyps (GP), and in differentiating malignant from benign causes in a select, homogeneous group of patients with 1- to 2-cm GPs. On visual assessment, 80% of malignant GPs and 20% of benign GPs had FDG uptake higher than normal liver uptake. The investigators found that all parameters derived from FDG uptake, especially the GP-to-liver uptake ratio of 1.14, constituted a strong risk factor that can be used to more effectively determine the necessity of surgical intervention than other known risk factors such as age, sex, presence of gallstone, and GP size.

Pancreas

Both benign and malignant disease of the pancreas can have a spectrum of FDG avidity.[61] For example, both pancreatic adenocarcinoma (the most common primary pancreatic malignancy) and pancreatitis (the most common primary pancreatic inflammatory condition) can be either intensely FDG-avid or only minimally FDG-avid, owing in part to the extent of disease, inflammation, fibrosis, and/or cystic components. Moreover, pancreatic disease can be difficult to characterize accurately on noncontrast CT, and pancreatic abnormalities are commonly evaluated with a multimodality imaging approach including contrast-enhanced CT and MR imaging.[62,63]

GI Tract

Increased FDG uptake in the GI tract can be due to inflammation, infection, or granulomatous disease. FDG-PET/CT can localize segments of inflamed bowel in patients with ulcers, inflammatory bowel disease, infectious colitis, diverticulitis, and hemorrhoids, among others. Research into the value of FDG-PET/CT as a noninvasive tool for evaluating Crohn's disease and/or ulcerative colitis is ongoing.[64] To avoid false-positive results, careful examination of the CT portion of the PET/CT study as well as clinical correlation is essential. Benign polyps in the GI tract are common incidental findings on FDG-PET/CT. Benign polyps can have several appearances and can be of different histologic subtypes. For example, polyps of the GI tract may be sessile or protrude into the bowel lumen. Hyperplastic and adenomatous polyps are the most common histologic subtypes. Hyperplastic polyps are typically not FDG-avid and do not have malignant transformation potential.[65] Adenomatous polyps can be mild to intensely FDG-avid, and have potential for malignant transformation with the likelihood of transformation increasing in relation to increasing size. In an article by Kamel and colleagues,[66] 39% of incidentally detected FDG-avid GI-tract nodules were adenomatous polyps. Incidentally detected adenomatous polyps are often larger than 10 mm,[67] although with improved resolution of PET/CT scanners smaller polyps can also be detected, particularly when these protrude into the bowel lumen.[68] Colonoscopy can be helpful for additional characterization when a colonic polyp is suspected, and provides the ability to remove a polyp found during the examination.

GU Tract

Detection of renal abnormalities are often a blind spot for PET. Both benign and malignant neoplasms may be minimally to intensely FDG-avid. For example, an oncocytoma (a benign renal neoplasm) often has FDG uptake comparable to that of normal renal parenchyma, and is indistinguishable from renal cell carcinoma on PET/CT. Moreover, intensely FDG-avid disease may be obscured by physiologic excreted FDG activity in the GU tract. Patients with equivocal renal findings on PET/CT can be referred for further evaluation with ultrasonography, contrast-enhanced CT, or MR imaging. Although ultrasonography and contrast-enhanced CT are commonly used, MR imaging has exquisite soft-tissue contrast and high sensitivity for small amounts of gadolinium-based contrast agents, making it the imaging modality of choice to detect solid/nodular enhancing components within cystic renal lesions or disease extension into the adjacent soft tissue/vascular structures.

SUMMARY

FDG-PET/CT is a powerful tool in the detection, staging, and follow-up of patients with carcinoma. Anatomic imaging alone is limited in detecting disease extent and response to therapy. The combination of metabolic and anatomic imaging provides a powerful tool, although image interpretation can be complicated by the large field of view, multiplicity of images that need to be reviewed, and conditions that cause increased FDG uptake. In particular, to ensure accurate FDG-PET/CT interpretation it is important to have an understanding of both normal and abnormal imaging appearances commonly encountered in oncology patients. This article discusses the commonly seen normal variations on FDG-PET/CT of the abdomen. To meet growing clinical and therapeutic needs, continued work is ongoing on standardization of imaging techniques, improved accessibility to accurate up-to-date clinical information, and increased availability of prior imaging.

REFERENCES

1. Engel H, Steinert H, Buck A, et al. Whole-body PET: physiological and artifactual fluorodeoxyglucose accumulations. J Nucl Med 1996;37:441–6.

2. Heusner TA, Hahn S, Hamami ME, et al. Gastrointestinal ^{18}F-FDG accumulation on PET without a corresponding CT abnormality is not an early indicator of cancer development. Eur Radiol 2009;19: 2171–9.

3. Jadvar H. Colonic FDG uptake pattern in subjects receiving oral contrast with no known or suspected colonic disease. Clin Nucl Med 2011;36:754–6.

4. Meisner RS, Spier BJ, Einarsson S, et al. Pilot study using PET/CT as a novel, noninvasive assessment of disease activity in inflammatory bowel disease. Inflamm Bowel Dis 2007;13:993–1000.

5. Ahn BC, Lee SW, Lee J. Intense accumulation of F-18 FDG in colonic wall in adult onset still disease with pseudomembranous colitis. Clin Nucl Med 2008;33:806–8.

6. Rubin DT, Surma BL, Gavzy SJ, et al. Positron emission tomography (PET) used to image subclinical inflammation associated with ulcerative colitis (UC) in remission. Inflamm Bowel Dis 2009;15: 750–5.

7. Tatlidil R, Jadvar H, Bading JR, et al. Incidental colonic fluorodeoxyglucose uptake: correlation with colonoscopic and histopathologic findings. Radiology 2002;224:783–7.

8. Gutman F, Alberini JL, Wartski M, et al. Incidental colonic focal lesions detected by FDG PET/CT. AJR Am J Roentgenol 2005;185:495–500.

9. Israel O, Yefremov N, Bar-Shalom R, et al. PET/CT detection of unexpected gastrointestinal foci of ^{18}F-FDG uptake: incidence, localization patterns, and clinical significance. J Nucl Med 2005;46: 758–62.

10. Lee JC, Hartnett GF, Hughes BG, et al. The segmental distribution and clinical significance of colorectal fluorodeoxyglucose uptake incidentally detected on PET-CT. Nucl Med Commun 2009;30: 333–7.

11. Gollub MJ, Akhurst TJ, Willamson MJ, et al. Feasibility of ex vivo FDG PET of the colon. Radiology 2009;252:232–9.

12. Zukotynski K, Lewis A, O'Regan K, et al. PET/CT and renal pathology: a blind spot for radiologists?

13. Zukotynski K, Lewis A, O'Regan K, et al. PET/CT and renal pathology: a blind spot for radiologists? Part 2—lymphoma, leukemia, and metastatic disease. AJR Am J Roentgenol 2012;199(2): W168–74.

14. Kubota K, Watanabe H, Murata Y, et al. Effects of blood glucose level on FDG uptake by liver: a FDG-PET/CT study. Nucl Med Biol 2011;38(3): 347–51.

15. Malladi A, Viner M, Jackson T, et al. PET/CT mediastinal and liver FDG uptake: effects of biological and procedural factors. J Med Imaging Radiat Oncol 2013;57(2):169–75.

16. Epelbaum R, Frenkel A, Haddad R, et al. Tumor aggressiveness and patient outcome in cancer of the pancreas assessed by dynamic ^{18}F-FDG PET/CT. J Nucl Med 2013;54(1):12–8.

17. Yun M, Kim W, Alnafisi N, et al. ^{18}F-FDG PET in characterizing adrenal lesions detected on CT or MRI. J Nucl Med 2001;42(12):1795–9.

18. Ozcan Kara P, Kara T, Kara Gedik G, et al. The role of fluorodeoxyglucose-positron emission tomography/computed tomography in differentiating between benign and malignant adrenal lesions. Nucl Med Commun 2011;32(2):106–12.

19. Boland GW, Dwamena BA, Jagtiani Singwaiya M, et al. Characterization of adrenal masses by using FDG PET: a systematic review and meta-analysis of diagnostic test performance. Radiology 2011; 259(1):117–26.

20. Miraldi F, Vesselle H, Faulhaber PF, et al. Elimination of artifactual accumulation of FDG in PET imaging of colorectal cancer. Clin Nucl Med 1998; 23:3–7.

21. Kamel EM, Jichlinski P, Prior JO, et al. Forced diuresis improves the diagnostic accuracy of ^{18}F-FDG PET in abdominopelvic malignancies. J Nucl Med 2006;47(11):1803–7.

22. Soyka JD, Strobel K, Veit-Haibach P, et al. Influence of bowel preparation before ^{18}F-FDG PET/CT on physiologic ^{18}F-FDG activity in the intestine. J Nucl Med 2010;51:507–10.

23. Murphy R, Doerger KM, Nathan MA, et al. Pretreatment with diphenoxylate hydrochloride/atropine sulfate (Lomotil) does not decrease physiologic bowel FDG activity on PET/CT scans of the abdomen and pelvis. Mol Imaging Biol 2009;11:114–7.

24. Jadvar H, Schambye RB, Segall GM. Effect of atropine and sincalide on the intestinal uptake of F-18 fluorodeoxyglucose. Clin Nucl Med 1999;24:965–7.

25. SNMMI practice guidelines. Available at: http:// interactive.snm.org/index.cfm?PageID=772. Accessed May 26, 2013.

26. Nayak B, Dogra PN, Naswa N, et al. Diuretic ^{18}F-FDG PET/CT imaging for detection and

locoregional staging of urinary bladder cancer: prospective evaluation of a novel technique. Eur J Nucl Med Mol Imaging 2013;40(3):386–93.

27. Anjos DA, Etchebehere EC, Ramos CD, et al. ^{18}F-FDG PET/CT delayed images after diuretic for restaging invasive bladder cancer. J Nucl Med 2007;48(5):764–70.

28. Otsuka H, Kubo A, Graham M, et al. The relationship between standard uptake value (SUV) and Hounsfield unit (HU) of oral contrast agent for FDG PET/CT study. J Med Invest 2004;51:226–9.

29. Cohade C, Osman M, Nakamoto Y, et al. Initial experience with oral contrast in PET/CT: phantom and clinical studies. J Nucl Med 2003;44:412–6.

30. Otero HJ, Yap JT, Patak MA, et al. Evaluation of low-density neutral oral contrast material in PET/CT for tumor imaging: results of a randomized clinical trial. AJR Am J Roentgenol 2009; 193(2):326–32.

31. Chun H, Kim CK, Krynckyi BR, et al. The usefulness of a repeat study for differentiating between bowel activity and local tumor recurrence on FDG PET scans. Clin Nucl Med 2003;28:672–3.

32. Massollo M, Marini C, Brignone M, et al. Metformin temporal and localized effects on gut glucose metabolism assessed using ^{18}F-FDG PET in mice. J Nucl Med 2013;54:259–66.

33. Gontier E, Fourme E, Wartski M, et al. High and typical ^{18}F-FDG bowel uptake in patients treated with metformin. Eur J Nucl Med Mol Imaging 2008;35:95–9.

34. Bybel B, Greenberg D, Paterson J, et al. Increased F-18 intestinal uptake in diabetic patients on metformin: a matched case-control analysis. Clin Nucl Med 2011;36(6):452–6.

35. Oh JR, Song HC, Chong A, et al. Impact of medication discontinuation on increased intestinal FDG accumulation in diabetic patients treated with metformin. AJR Am J Roentgenol 2010;195:1404–10.

36. Ozülker T, Ozülker F, Mert M, et al. Clearance of the high intestinal (18)F-FDG uptake associated with metformin after stopping the drug. Eur J Nucl Med Mol Imaging 2010;37:1011–7.

37. Yao WJ, Hoh CK, Hawkins RA, et al. Quantitative PET imaging of bone marrow glucose metabolic response to hematopoietic cytokines. J Nucl Med 1995;36:794–9.

38. Knopp MV, Bischoff H, Rimac A, et al. Bone marrow uptake of fluorine-18-fluorodeoxyglucose following treatment with hematopoietic growth factors: initial evaluation. Nucl Med Biol 1996;23:845–9.

39. Sugawara Y, Fisher SJ, Zasadny KR, et al. Preclinical and clinical studies of bone marrow uptake of fluorine-18-fluorodeoxyglucose with or without granulocyte colony-stimulating factor during chemotherapy. J Clin Oncol 1998;16:173–80.

40. Hollinger EF, Alibazoglu H, Ali A, et al. Hematopoietic cytokine-mediated FDG uptake simulates the appearance of diffuse metastatic disease on whole-body PET imaging. Clin Nucl Med 1998;23:93–8.

41. Sugawara Y, Zasadny KR, Kison PV, et al. Splenic fluorodeoxyglucose uptake increased by granulocyte colony-stimulating factor therapy: PET imaging results. J Nucl Med 1999;40(9):1456–62.

42. Pak K, Kim SJ, Kim IJ, et al. Impact of cytokines on diffuse splenic ^{18}F-fluorodeoxyglucose uptake during positron emission tomography/computed tomography. Nucl Med Commun 2013; 34(1):64–70.

43. Gessner K. Conradi Gesneri Medici Tigurini Historiae Animalium: Lib 1-De Quadrupedibus Viviparis (1551).

44. Kim S, Krynyckyi BR, Machac J, et al. Temporal relation between temperature change and FDG uptake in brown adipose tissue. Eur J Nucl Med Mol Imaging 2008;35:984–9.

45. Cannon B, Nedergaard J. Brown adipose tissue: function and physiological significance. Physiol Rev 2004;84:277–359.

46. Garcia CA, Van Nostrand D, Atkins F, et al. Reduction of brown fat 2-deoxy-2-[F-18] fluoro-D-glucose uptake by controlling environmental temperature prior to positron emission tomography scan. Mol Imaging Biol 2006;8:24–9.

47. Christensen CR, Clark PB, Morton KA. Reversal of hypermetabolic brown adipose tissue in F-18 FDG PET imaging. Clin Nucl Med 2006;31:193–6.

48. Garcia CA, Van Nostrand D, Majd M, et al. Benzodiazepine-resistant "brown fat" pattern in positron emission tomography: two case reports of resolution with temperature control. Mol Imaging Biol 2004;6:368–72.

49. Zukotynski KA, Fahey FH, Laffin S, et al. Seasonal variation in the effect of constant ambient temperature of 24 degrees C in reducing FDG uptake by brown adipose tissue in children. Eur J Nucl Med Mol Imaging 2010;37(10):1854–60.

50. Zukotynski KA, Fahey FH, Laffin S, et al. Constant ambient temperature of 24 degrees C significantly reduces FDG uptake by brown adipose tissue in children scanned during the winter. Eur J Nucl Med Mol Imaging 2009;36(4):602–6.

51. Gelfand MJ, O'Hara SM, Curtwright LA, et al. Premedication to block [(18)F]FDG uptake in the brown adipose tissue of pediatric and adolescent patients. Pediatr Radiol 2005;35:984–90.

52. Parysow O, Mollerach AM, Jager V, et al. Low-dose oral propranolol could reduce brown adipose tissue F-18 FDG uptake in patients undergoing PET scans. Clin Nucl Med 2007;32:351–7.

53. Söderlund V, Larsson SA, Jacobsson H. Reduction of FDG uptake in brown adipose tissue in clinical

patients by a single dose of propranolol. Eur J Nucl Med Mol Imaging 2007;34:1018–22.

54. Tatsumi M, Engles JM, Ishimori T, et al. Intense (18) F-FDG uptake in brown adipose fat can be reduced pharmacologically. J Nucl Med 2004;45: 1189–93.

55. Williams G, Kolodny GM. Method for decreasing uptake of ^{18}F-FDG by hypermetabolic brown adipose tissue on PET. AJR Am J Roentgenol 2008; 190(5):1406–9.

56. Delbeke D, Martin WH, Sandler MP, et al. Evaluation of benign vs malignant hepatic lesions with positron emission tomography. Arch Surg 1998; 133:510–5.

57. Iwata Y, Shiomi S, Sasaki N, et al. Clinical usefulness of positron emission tomography with fluorine-18-fluorodeoxyglucose in the diagnosis of liver tumors. Ann Nucl Med 2000;14(2):121–6.

58. Sumiyoshi T, Moriguchi M, Kanemoto H, et al. Liver-specific contrast agent-enhanced magnetic resonance and ^{18}F-fluorodeoxyglucose positron emission tomography findings of hepatocellular adenoma: report of a case. Surg Today 2012;42:200–4.

59. Aznar DL, Ojeda R, Garcia EU, et al. Focal nodular hyperplasia (FNH): a potential cause of false-positive positron emission tomography. Clin Nucl Med 2005;30(9):636–7.

60. Lee J, Yun M, Kim KS, et al. Risk stratification of gallbladder polyps (1-2 cm) for surgical intervention with ^{18}F-FDG PET/CT. J Nucl Med 2012;53: 353–8.

61. Sahani DV, Bonaffini P, Catalano O, et al. State-of-the-art PET/CT of the pancreas: current role and emerging indications. Radiographics 2012;32(4): 1133–58.

62. Buchs NC, Bühler L, Bucher P, et al. Value of contrast-enhanced ^{18}F-fluorodeoxyglucose positron emission tomography/computed tomography in detection and presurgical assessment of pancreatic cancer: a prospective study. J Gastroenterol Hepatol 2011;26(4):657–62.

63. Michl P, Pauls S, Gress TM. Evidence-based diagnosis and staging of pancreatic cancer. Best Pract Res Clin Gastroenterol 2006;20(2):227–51.

64. Löffler M, Weckesser M, Franzius C, et al. High diagnostic value of ^{18}F-FDG-PET in pediatric patients with chronic inflammatory bowel disease. Ann N Y Acad Sci 2006;1072:379–85.

65. Abdel-Nabi H, Doerr RJ, Lamonica DM, et al. Staging of primary colorectal carcinomas with fluorine-18 fluorodeoxyglucose whole-body PET: correlation with histopathologic and CT findings. Radiology 1998;206(3):755–60.

66. Kamel EM, Thumshirn M, Truninger K, et al. Significance of incidental ^{18}F-FDG accumulations in the gastrointestinal tract in PET/CT: correlation with endoscopic and histopathologic results. J Nucl Med 2004;45(11):1804–10.

67. Yasuda S, Fujii H, Nakahara T, et al. ^{18}F-FDG PET detection of colonic adenomas. J Nucl Med 2001; 42(7):989–92.

68. Gollub MJ, Akhurst T, Markowitz AJ, et al. Combined CT colonography and ^{18}F-FDG PET of colon polyps: potential technique for selective detection of cancer and precancerous lesions. AJR Am J Roentgenol 2007;188(1):130–8.

Pelvis
Normal Variants and Benign Findings in FDG-PET/CT Imaging

Andres Kohan, MD[a,b], Norbert E. Avril, MD[a,*]

KEYWORDS

- FDG-PET • PET/CT • Benign findings • Pelvis • Normal variants

KEY POINTS

- In FDG-PET/CT, physiologic and benign incidental findings in the pelvis can occur in more than 1% of patients with cancer.
- It is important to interpret an incidental finding in the context of the underlying disease of the patient.
- CT images analyzed in different planes (axial, sagittal, and coronal) and different windows (bone, soft tissue, and so forth) often help to determine the nature of increased FDG uptake.
- In female premenopausal patients the menstrual cycle should be taken into account.
- If possible, incidental findings should be correlated with other imaging modalities, physical examination, and laboratory results for further characterization.

INTRODUCTION

Fluorodeoxyglucose (FDG)-PET/computed tomography (CT) has become one of the most important imaging modalities for patients with cancer. Therefore, when developing a potential differential diagnosis for increased FDG uptake, it is of crucial importance to consider benign conditions and normal variants, which can present with increased FDG accumulation, particularly in the pelvis. The CT portion of PET/CT often provides helpful information about the nature of incidental findings. This is becoming more relevant as an increasing number of FDG-PET/CT studies are performed with a full diagnostic, contrast-enhanced CT. Furthermore, normal variants and benign findings are also relevant when using FDG-PET/magnetic resonance (MR) imaging to assess the pelvis.

Studies have shown that increased FDG uptake in the pelvis is fairly common. For example, a study of oncologic patients found an incidence of at least 1.1% of isolated pelvic foci of increased FDG uptake not related to cancer.[1] The limited specificity of FDG-PET is well known because increased glucose metabolism is not a unique feature of cancer but is also seen in benign conditions, such as inflammation, granulomatous disease, benign adenomas, and endometriosis.[2–4] Nonetheless, FDG-PET provides a high sensitivity for identification and characterization of pelvic malignancies, requiring a profound understanding of FDG-avid benign conditions and potential pitfalls to derive a correct interpretation. Often anatomic imaging offers important information about a potential differential diagnosis. This includes the correct identification of metabolically active lymph nodes and FDG uptake within bowel structures, the ureters,

Conflict of Interest: The authors declare no conflict of interest.
 ^a Department of Radiology, Case Western Reserve University, University Hospitals Case Medical Center, 11100 Euclid Avenue, BSH 5056, Cleveland, OH 44106, USA; ^b Department of Radiology, Hospital Italiano de Buenos Aires, Juan D. Peron 4190, C1181ACH, Ciudad Autónoma de Buenos Aires, Argentina
* Corresponding author. Department of Radiology, Case Western Reserve University, University Hospitals Case Medical Center, 11100 Euclid Avenue, BSH 5056, Cleveland, OH 44106.
E-mail address: Norbert.Avril@case.edu

PET Clin 9 (2014) 185–193
http://dx.doi.org/10.1016/j.cpet.2013.10.002
1556-8598/14/$ – see front matter © 2014 Elsevier Inc. All rights reserved.

the ovaries, and the osseous structures. This article describes the most common benign findings and normal variations in the pelvis that could lead to false-positive findings in FDG-PET/CT.

Bone Benign Pathology

On many occasions bone lesions can be seen on FDG-PET/CT. Although the association of bony lesions to the presence of increased FDG uptake might indicate tumor involvement, it might also be related to a benign condition, such as Paget disease, fibrous dysplasia, osteoarthritis, or insufficiency fractures. It is therefore important to take the CT appearances of hypermetabolic abnormalities into account.

Paget disease involves abnormal bone destruction and remodeling. Most patients have no specific symptoms, although occasionally bone pain is present, which in oncologic patients would raise concerns for metastasis. Paget disease usually affects one or more areas of the skeleton, with the pelvis as a frequent site of involvement. It is usually diagnosed through plain film radiographs or a CT scan performed for other reasons. Bone scintigraphy is a sensitive method showing the extent of bone remodeling. On FDG-PET/CT, lesions can demonstrate increased FDG uptake depending on the stage of disease[5,6] because Paget pathophysiology is divided in phases that likely have different glycolytic activity. The CT component of PET/CT typically shows areas of osteolysis, cortical thickening and sclerosis, or both in the affected bone, often in an asymmetric pattern. Some studies have shown the usefulness of FDG-PET/CT to monitor the treatment of Paget disease.[7]

Fibrous dysplasia of the bone is a benign nonhereditary and relatively common bone disease characterized by replacement of normal bone with abnormal fibro-osseous tissue. This is caused by the inability of the bone-forming elements to produce mature lamellar bone. As in Paget disease, fibrous dysplasia is usually asymptomatic but can occasionally cause bone pain, and is often incidentally identified on imaging studies performed for other reasons. On CT, the lesions are usually well defined, intramedullary in location, and expansile. Variable bone density is seen within lesions with areas of ground-glass opacity and a sclerotic rim. Increased glucose metabolism by fibrous dysplasia is well documented.[8] Interestingly, fibrous dysplasia also shows increased choline metabolism, which can be seen when using [C-11]Choline[9] for imaging prostate cancer.

Osteoarthritis has been suggested to reflect an age-related dynamic reaction pattern of joints

in response to insult or injury.[10] This often results in an inflammatory reaction and subsequently increased FDG uptake, often visualized within the hip joint. CT images generally guide the diagnosis, because increased FDG uptake can be localized to the hip joint with typical degenerative changes seen on CT.

Insufficiency fractures are similar to stress fractures caused by normal efforts placed on weakened bone, which present with increased FDG uptake. Patients with a known history of pelvic radiotherapy have a higher incidence of insufficiency fractures, reported to be between 8.2% and 19.7%.[11] When using bone scintigraphy, a characteristic "H pattern" caused by fractures of both sacral alae and a horizontal component involving the sacral body has been reported to be highly sensitive and specific, whereas the absence of the "H pattern" reduces the specificity.[11] MR imaging has also proved sensitive and specific for identifying insufficiency fractures, whereas CT is less sensitive compared with bone scintigraphy or MR imaging.[12]

It is important to consider malignant fractures as a differential diagnosis. In malignant fractures increased FDG uptake in the bone marrow is usually present, whereas the bone marrow is usually not metabolically active in benign fractures.[11] Although the use of standardized uptake value has been suggested in the literature to aid in the differential diagnosis, no definite evidence currently exists to support its ability to differentiate between benign or malignant bone lesions.[6]

Colon Benign Pathology

On FDG-PET/CT images there are usually two patterns of increased FDG uptake that can be seen in the colon: focal and diffuse. Diffusely increased FDG uptake is usually related to smooth muscle activity or intraluminal excretion and accumulation; intensely increased FDG uptake within the bowel is sometimes related to medication used for treatment of diabetes mellitus (eg, metformin).[13] However, focal FDG uptake raises concern for neoplastic, preneoplastic, or inflammatory disease (**Fig. 1**). It is important to point out that focally increased FDG uptake, particularly when related to a potential mass on CT, should be considered suspicious for malignancy. Reports evaluating the incidence and clinical significance of incidental FDG uptake in the colon concluded that appropriate follow-up investigations should be performed.[14]

Focal colonic FDG uptake can also be seen in polyps. Colonic polyps are benign lesions with malignant potential. The risk of cancer in an individual

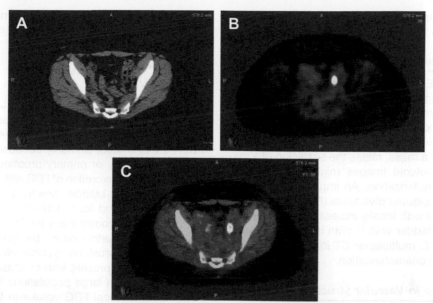

Fig. 1. (A) CT image of sigmoid colon. Focal FDG uptake in the sigmoid colon visualized by FDG-PET (B) and fusion images (C). The CT image (A) shows no focal thickening of the colonic wall and the pericolonic fat remains unaltered indicating that this finding is probably benign in origin. A colonoscopy did not reveal a relevant finding.

polyp is related to its histologic type and the size and degree of cellular atypia. Studies that have investigated the relationship between focal FDG uptake and the presence of lesions found on colonoscopy concluded that FDG-PET/CT has a high sensitivity but low specificity for cancer because most of the metabolically active lesions corresponded to polyps.[4] Nonetheless, this is still of clinical relevance because polyps are known preneoplastic lesions that can further develop into cancer. The degree of FDG uptake seen on PET also depends on the size of lesions,[15] and it is often more difficult to identify lesions in close proximity to the bladder.

Another colonic benign pathology with increased FDG uptake is diverticulitis. Colonic diverticulosis is quite common among the elderly population in which colon cancer is also more frequent. Colonic diverticulosis often is not composed of true diverticula but rather outpouchings of colonic mucosa caused by increased intraluminal pressure, thus lacking the three layers of the colonic wall. Diverticulosis is more common in the western population than in Asia, probably because of a difference in the intake of dietary fiber. Anatomic localization of diverticulosis is most commonly in the sigmoid colon. Out of the 70% of patients older than 70 years of age that have diverticulosis, 20% may experience an inflammatory complication.[16] In these patients focal or segmental FDG uptake

caused by diverticulitis might be present in the pelvis. It is important to consider that colonic stenosis caused by a chronic inflammatory process has also been reported to present with increased FDG uptake.[17] It is therefore necessary to know the CT characteristics of these findings. Absence of eccentric wall thickening, a luminal mass, or enlarged pericolonic lymph nodes in the presence of diverticulosis favor an inflammatory cause particularly when accompanied with inflammation or edema and fluid in the root of the mesentery.[18] Distribution of FDG uptake related to the bowel rather than focally is also suggestive of a benign cause. A report in which increased FDG uptake secondary to diverticulitis was seen initially but absent on a delayed PET acquisition[19] could suggest that dual time point PET imaging might be helpful in determining the cause of colonic uptake in the pelvis. However, dual time point PET imaging is not generally accepted and larger-scale prospective studies are yet to be conducted.

Appendicitis has also been reported as a possible false-positive finding when staging for cancer presenting with increased FDG uptake.[20] Although in young patients appendicitis is usually accompanied by a typical clinical presentation, in older patients' appendicitis might be present without specific signs or symptoms. Nonetheless, primary appendicular cancer has a reported incidence of 0.08%[20] and is therefore less likely.

Typical CT appearances of the latter can include a cystic mass with mural nodules.

Bladder Benign Pathology

Although PET/CT is not considered standard of care for staging of patients with bladder cancer, urothelial tumors and metastatic lymph nodes present with increased FDG uptake.[21] Hence focal uptake within the bladder wall, particularly in the presence of a mass, raises the suspicion of a malignancy. Postvoid images might be helpful for further characterization. An important differential diagnosis is bladder diverticula (**Fig. 2**), which typically present with focally increased FDG retention within the bladder wall.[21] With the current use of multislice CT, multiplanar CT images often allow for accurate characterization.

FDG Uptake in Vascular Structures

Both iliac arteries are subject to the same pathologic processes as other large vessels, particularly atherosclerotic plaques, which can appear as areas of focally increased FDG uptake.[22,23] Pathologic processes in iliac veins include thrombosis, which can also present with increased FDG uptake.[24] A deep vein thrombosis can also become infected resulting in moderate to intensely increased FDG uptake localized within vessels and surrounding tissues.[25]

Both atherosclerotic plaques and deep vein thrombosis can be further evaluated by contrast-enhanced CT demonstrating a stenosis in the case of an atherosclerotic plaque or occlusion of a vessel in the case of thrombosis.

MALE PELVIS
Prostate Benign Pathology

Prostate cancer is the second most common neoplasia among men. However, detection with FDG-PET is limited, primarily because of the low metabolic activity of primary prostate cancer. In addition, urinary excretion of FDG with high urinary activity within the bladder directly adjacent to the prostate gland and focal activity retention within the urethra can compromise the interpretation of PET images. Furthermore, benign pathology, such as benign prostatic hyperplasia and prostatitis (**Fig. 3**), can present with increased FDG uptake.[26] Studies in large populations have shown that incidental focal FDG uptake in the prostate can be secondary to cancer in 0.05% to 19.2% of the cases,[26] depending on the initial indication for PET imaging (patients with benign diseases vs patients with cancer). The level of FDG uptake does not allow further characterization of increased FDG uptake as benign or malignant. Some reports have suggested that FDG uptake in a marginal location of the peripheral part of the gland seems to be more concerning for malignancy.[27] In summary, even though focal uptake can be seen in benign conditions, such as benign prostatic hyperplasia and prostatitis, if associated

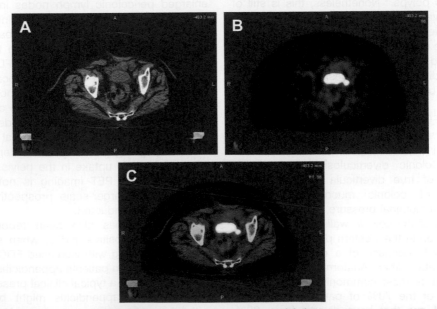

Fig. 2. Bladder diverticula on CT (*A*), FDG-PET (*B*), and fusion images (*C*) that initially suggested the presence of a hypermetabolic lymph node next to the bladder on axial images. Further assessment in the sagittal and coronal planes identified the finding as benign.

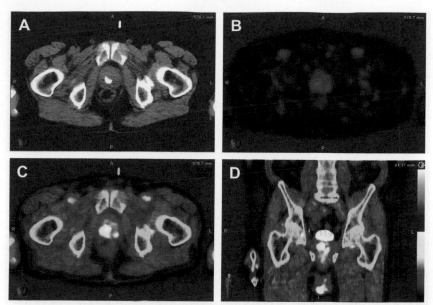

Fig. 3. (A) CT image shows an enlarged prostate gland with calcifications. FDG-PET (B) and fusion images (C, D) demonstrate focal FDG uptake in the medial aspect of the prostate gland. Digital examination and prostate-specific antigen level support the benign cause.

with high prostate-specific antigen values or other abnormal findings an ultrasound-guided biopsy might be warranted.

Male Reproductive System

Increased accumulation of FDG in the testicles has been documented and studied in a relatively small number of cases.[28–30] There is often physiologically mild increased FDG uptake, which has been related to facilitated glucose transport in Leydig cells for testosterone production.[30] Another possible explanation is the presence of increased expression of Glut 3 in Sertoli cells and early spermatocytes.[29] Of note, an undescended or ascended testicle should be considered when a "mass" is present in the inguinal canal presenting with increased FDG accumulation.[31] Confusion with lymph node involvement has been reported.[31]

Other clinical conditions, such as infections, could prompt a false-positive finding because of increased FDG uptake; however, such circumstances are probably rare because of the symptoms associated.

FEMALE PELVIS
Normal Variants

Generally, in postmenopausal women the female pelvic organs, including the ovaries and the uterus, demonstrate low metabolic activity.[32] In premenopausal women, however, there is a variable degree of increased FDG uptake seen within the ovaries,

usually unilaterally, between the 10th and 25th day of the menstrual cycle. Peak uptake is often at the time of ovulation with focally increased FDG accumulation in a spherical or discoid form, showing smooth margins on CT. Yun and colleagues[33] reported the presence of physiologic bilateral increased FDG uptake during the ovulatory or periovulatory phase in the adnexal area, corresponding to uptake of the fallopian tubes, in 8.8% of their study population. The authors recommended taking the menstrual cycle into account to determine the origin of positive incidental findings. It has also been reported that a luteal cyst can present with increased FDG accumulation.[34]

The uterus can show physiologic mild, diffusely increased FDG uptake within the endometrium during midcycle (**Fig. 4**) and intracavity activity retention during menstruation.[32] Uterine physiologic uptake was studied in relationship to muscle contractions during menstrual and nonmenstrual periods assessed by cine MR imaging[35] with no convincing relationship observed.

Although pregnancy is a contraindication for imaging studies that involve radiation, a patient might be unaware of an early pregnancy. There are a few case reports exemplifying an early pregnancy in FDG-PET/CT, and in one of those it was demonstrated that FDG crosses the placental barrier and accumulates in fetal tissue.[36] Meanwhile, there was mild increased placental FDG uptake in one case[37] and no increased FDG uptake in a second case.[36]

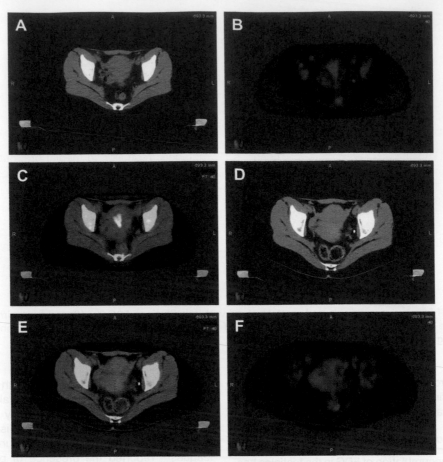

Fig. 4. A 43-year-old patient studied with FDG-PET/CT on two different days of her menstrual cycle. CT images (*A, D*) show no findings suggesting active pelvic disease, although the sensitivity of non-contrast CT is low for pelvic organs. Increased endometrial FDG uptake is seen in the axial plane with a typical triangular shape of the endometrium on FDG-PET (*B, C*). The absence of increased FDG uptake in the study performed at a later date (*E, F*) confirms the benign origin of this finding.

Uterine Benign Pathology

Uterine leiomyomas have an incidence of 30% in fertile women, and can develop long before menopause. Leiomyomas often present with mild increased FDG uptake, although intense FDG uptake can occasionally be seen, more frequently in premenopausal woman than in the postmenopause period. Degenerated leiomyomas are generally characterized by high signal intensity on T2-weighted sequences on MR imaging and often have higher FDG uptake than those showing low signal intensity on T2-weighted images.[38] Increased FDG uptake occurs in 0.1% of healthy women, 0.5% of women with known leiomyomas, and 3.4% of women with degenerated leiomyomas.[39] Correlation with anatomic imaging, particularly ultrasound or MR imaging, is often helpful and in cases with intensely increased FDG uptake a

leiomyosarcoma should be considered. Uterine leiomyosarcoma is infrequent accounting for 1% to 3% of all uterine cancers. Nonetheless, because of its highly aggressive behavior and frequent recurrence, it accounts for 15% of uterine malignancy-related deaths.

Another benign condition that can cause increased FDG uptake is the presence of adenomyosis or endometriosis. Adenomyosis is a common nonneoplastic gynecologic disease characterized by excessive migration of the endometrial glands and stroma from the basal layer of the endometrium into the myometrium.[40] This often results in inflammatory changes and hormone-dependent changes of the myometrium resulting in false-positives findings.[40] In these cases CT is not very helpful for further characterization, because adenomyosis is usually diagnosed by the thickness of junctional zone of the uterus or changes in the myometrium. Endovaginal ultrasound can be helpful but the imaging modality of choice is MR imaging.[41]

The presence of an intrauterine contraceptive device (IUD) can be a source of increased FDG uptake.[42] This is probably related to the presence of an inflammatory response to the IUD, which is believed to have a role in the contraceptive effectiveness.[43] Copper-based IUDs are easily seen on CT; other types of IUDs are often better visualized with endovaginal ultrasound. References to the existence of an IUD might also be found in the medical record of the patient.

Adnexal Benign Pathology

FDG-PET and PET/CT provide a high sensitivity for detecting adnexal tumors but have a low specificity because of inflammatory processes or benign tumors.[44] The level of FDG uptake including the use of standardized uptake value does not allow the differentiation between an acute inflammatory process and ovarian malignancy.[45] Also, there are several benign tumors of the ovary, such as mature teratomas,[45] endometriomas,[46] fibromas or fibrothecomas,[46] and Brenner tumors,[47] which can present with increased FDG uptake.

Mature teratomas can demonstrate moderately increased FDG uptake, which is often nonspecific,[46] but mature teratomas are easily identifiable on CT, ultrasound, or MR imaging because of their imaging characteristics. Mature teratomas characteristically present mature tissue from the three germ layers (endoderm, ectoderm, and mesoderm), so it can frequently demonstrate hair, teeth, bone, and fat.

Endometriomas are cystic tumors of the ovaries that develop from endometrial implants on the ovaries and are filled with blood components and endometrial tissue, which can present with mild increased FDG uptake.[46] Endometriomas are usually correctly identified as cystic lesions on ultrasound containing echogenic material and on MR imaging showing T2 shading or hyperintensity on T1-weighted sequences.[48] Of note, malignant tumors may arise from an endometrioma (clear cell and endometrioid carcinoma) or coexist with them, so further assessment of those lesions should be made using other imaging methods when incidentally found on FDG-PET/CT.

Fibromas or fibrothecomas are the most common solid primary tumors of the ovary comprising 4% of all ovarian tumors. Unlike other ovarian tumors they evolve from gonadal stromal cells, and although the fibroma component is composed of dense fibrous tissue (hypoechogenic in ultrasound

or low signal in T2-weighted MR imaging), the stromal component is composed of lipid-rich laden cells. Their solid appearance can change as they increase in size with edematous or cystic degenerative changes. This would translate into a more heterogeneous aspect and higher T2-weighted signal in MR imaging. In about 40% of the cases, fibromas or fibrothecomas are associated with ascites, which is the main confounding factor when determining their origin.

Brenner tumors compose 2% to 3% of all ovarian neoplasms and are of epithelial origin. Although usually detected incidentally, they can occasionally cause symptoms, such as a palpable mass or pain. They usually present as a multilocular cystic mass with dense fibrous solid components, hence having low signal intensity on T2-weighted MR imaging sequences. Calcification within the solid component is a frequent finding. The difficulty of these imaging characteristics is that mucinous ovarian tumors can show calcifications, cystic components, and low-grade FDG uptake.

Other adnexal benign pathologies that are associated with increased FDG uptake are inflammatory or infectious conditions. Increased FDG uptake caused by infectious diseases, such as salpingitis, salpingo-oophoritis, or ovarian abscesses, has been reported.[45] In such cases the patient's clinical history, laboratory findings, and physical examination often help to determine the origin of the increased FDG uptake.

Superficial and deep peritoneal endometriosis is another cause for false-positive FDG uptake. However, although there are several reports describing endometriosis as a cause of false-positives in FDG-PET,[49] Fastrez and colleagues[50] found normal levels of FDG uptake in 10 out of 10 patients with known endometriosis, even in advanced stages of the disease or in the presence of severe symptoms.

REFERENCES

1. Khademi S, Westphalen AC, Webb EM, et al. Frequency and etiology of solitary hot spots in the pelvis at whole-body positron emission tomography/computed tomography imaging. Clin Imaging 2009;33(1):44–8.

2. De Gaetano AM, Calcagni ML, Rufini V, et al. Imaging of gynecologic malignancies with FDG PET-CT: case examples, physiologic activity, and pitfalls. Abdom Imaging 2009;34(6):696–711.

3. Metser U, Miller E, Lerman H, et al. Benign nonphysiologic lesions with increased 18F-FDG uptake on PET/CT: characterization and incidence. AJR Am J Roentgenol 2007;189(5):1203–10.

4. Roh SH, Jung SA, Kim SE, et al. The clinical meaning of benign colon uptake in (18)F-FDG PET: comparison with colonoscopic findings. Clin Endosc 2012;45(2):145–50.

5. Mahmood S, Martinez de Llano SR. Paget disease of the humerus mimicking metastatic disease in a patient with metastatic malignant mesothelioma on whole body F-18 FDG PET/CT. Clin Nucl Med 2008;33(7):510–2.

6. Mena LM, Hernandez AC, Gallego M, et al. Incidental detection of Paget disease on (18)F-FDG PET/CT scan in a patient with rectal cancer. Rev Esp Med Nucl Imagen Mol 2012;32(2):117–8 [in Spanish].

7. Installe J, Nzeusseu A, Bol A, et al. (18)F-fluoride PET for monitoring therapeutic response in Paget's disease of bone. J Nucl Med 2005;46(10):1650–8.

8. Su MG, Tian R, Fan QP, et al. Recognition of fibrous dysplasia of bone mimicking skeletal metastasis on 18F-FDG PET/CT imaging. Skeletal Radiol 2011; 40(3):295–302.

9. Gu CN, Hunt CH, Lehman VT, et al. Benign fibrous dysplasia on [(11)C]choline PET: a potential mimicker of disease in patients with biochemical recurrence of prostate cancer. Ann Nucl Med 2012; 26(7):599–602.

10. Busija L, Bridgett L, Williams SR, et al. Osteoarthritis. Best Pract Res Clin Rheumatol 2010;24(6): 757–68.

11. Park SH, Kim JC, Lee JE, et al. Pelvic insufficiency fracture after radiotherapy in patients with cervical cancer in the era of PET/CT. Radiat Oncol J 2011; 29(4):269–76.

12. Krestan C, Hojreh A. Imaging of insufficiency fractures. Eur J Radiol 2009;71(3):398–405.

13. Gontier E, Fourme E, Wartski M, et al. High and typical 18F-FDG bowel uptake in patients treated with metformin. Eur J Nucl Med Mol Imaging 2008;35(1):95–9.

14. Treglia G, Calcagni ML, Rufini V, et al. Clinical significance of incidental focal colorectal (18)F-fluorodeoxyglucose uptake: our experience and a review of the literature. Colorectal Dis 2012; 14(2):174–80.

15. Farquharson AL, Chopra A, Ford A, et al. Incidental focal colonic lesions found on (18)F-fluorodeoxyglucose positron emission tomography/computed tomography scan: further support for a national guideline on definitive management. Colorectal Dis 2012;14(2):e56–63.

16. Sheth AA, Longo W, Floch MH. Diverticular disease and diverticulitis. Am J Gastroenterol 2008;103(6): 1550–6.

17. Nishiyama N, Mori H, Kobara H, et al. Difficulty in differentiating two cases of sigmoid stenosis by diverticulitis from cancer. World J Gastroenterol 2012;10(27):3623–6.

18. Chintapalli KN, Chopra S, Ghiatas AA, et al. Diverticulitis versus colon cancer: differentiation with helical CT findings. Radiology 1999;210(2): 429–35.

19. Shen YY, Kao CH, Yeh LH, et al. Vanishing spot on dual-time-point FDG PET/CT: colonic diverticulitis. Clin Nucl Med 2010;35(7):529–31.

20. Ogawa S, Itabashi M, Kameoka S. Significance of FDG-PET in Identification of diseases of the appendix: based on experience of two cases falsely positive for FDG accumulation. Case Rep Gastroenterol 2009;3(1):125–30.

21. Lee ST, Lawrentschuk N, Scott AM. PET in prostate and bladder tumors. Semin Nucl Med 2012;42(4): 231–46.

22. Rudd JH, Myers KS, Bansilal S, et al. Relationships among regional arterial inflammation, calcification, risk factors, and biomarkers: a prospective fluorodeoxyglucose positron-emission tomography/computed tomography imaging study. Circ Cardiovasc Imaging 2009;2(2):107–15.

23. Bucci M, Aparici CM, Hawkins R, et al. Validation of FDG Uptake in the arterial wall as an imaging biomarker of atherosclerotic plaques with (18) F-fluorodeoxyglucose positron emission tomography-computed tomography (FDG-PET/CT). J Neuroimaging 2012 Aug 28. http://dx.doi.org/10.1111/j.1552-6569.2012.00740.x [Epub ahead of print] PubMed PMID: 22928741.

24. Rondina MT, Lam UT, Pendleton RC, et al. (18)F-FDG PET in the evaluation of acuity of deep vein thrombosis. Clin Nucl Med 2012;37(12):1139–45.

25. Miceli M, Atoui R, Walker R, et al. Diagnosis of deep septic thrombophlebitis in cancer patients by fluorine-18 fluorodeoxyglucose positron emission tomography scanning: a preliminary report. J Clin Oncol 2004;22(10):1949–56.

26. Hwang I, Chong A, Jung SI, et al. Is further evaluation needed for incidental focal uptake in the prostate in 18-fluoro-2-deoxyglucose positron emission tomography–computed tomography images? Ann Nucl Med 2013;27(2):140–5.

27. Han EJ, H O J, Choi WH, et al. Significance of incidental focal uptake in prostate on 18-fluoro-2-deoxyglucose positron emission tomography CT images. Br J Radiol 2010;83(995):915–20.

28. Goethals I, De Vriendt C, Hoste P, et al. Normal uptake of F-18 FDG in the testis as assessed by PET/CT in a pediatric study population. Ann Nucl Med 2009; 23(9):817–20.

29. Dierickx LO, Huyghe E, Nogueira D, et al. Functional testicular evaluation using PET/CT with 18F-fluorodeoxyglucose. Eur J Nucl Med Mol Imaging 2012;39(1):129–37.

30. Kitajima K, Nakamoto Y, Senda M, et al. Normal uptake of 18F-FDG in the testis: an assessment by PET/CT. Ann Nucl Med 2007;21(7):405–10.

31. Groheux D, Teyton P, Vercellino L, et al. Cryptorchidism as a potential source of misinterpretation in (18)FDG-PET imaging in restaging lymphoma patients. Biomed Pharmacother 2013;67(6):533–8.

32. Liu Y. Benign ovarian and endometrial uptake on FDG PET-CT: patterns and pitfalls. Ann Nucl Med 2009;23(2):107–12.

33. Yun M, Cho A, Lee JH, et al. Physiologic 18F-FDG uptake in the fallopian tubes at mid cycle on PET/CT. J Nucl Med 2010;51(5):682–5.

34. Bagga S. A corpus luteal cyst masquerading as a lymph node mass on PET/CT scan in a pregnant woman with an anterior mediastinal lymphomatous mass. Clin Nucl Med 2007;32(8):649–51.

35. Kido A, Nakamoto Y, Nishizawa S, et al. Physiological uptake of 18F-fluorodeoxyglucose in uterine endometrium and myometrium: correlation with uterine motility evaluated by cine magnetic resonance imaging. Acta Radiol 2009;50(4):455–61.

36. Zanotti-Fregonara P, Jan S, Taieb D, et al. Absorbed 18F-FDG dose to the fetus during early pregnancy. J Nucl Med 2010;51(5):803–5.

37. Zanotti-Fregonara P, Jan S, Champion C, et al. In vivo quantification of 18f-fdg uptake in human placenta during early pregnancy. Health Phys 2009;97(1):82–5.

38. Nishizawa S, Inubushi M, Kido A, et al. Incidence and characteristics of uterine leiomyomas with FDG uptake. Ann Nucl Med 2008;22(9):803–10.

39. Tsukada H, Murakami M, Shida M, et al. 18F-fluorodeoxyglucose uptake in uterine leiomyomas in healthy women. Clin Imaging 2009;33(6):462–7.

40. Yu JI, Huh SJ, Kim YI, et al. Variable uterine uptake of FDG in adenomyosis during concurrent chemoradiation therapy for cervical cancer. Radiat Oncol J 2011;29(3):214–7.

41. Reinhold C, Tafazoli F, Mehio A, et al. Uterine adenomyosis: endovaginal US and MR imaging features with histopathologic correlation. Radiographics 1999;19:S147–60.

42. Julian A, Payoux P, Rimailho J, et al. Uterine uptake of F-18 FDG on positron emission tomography induced by an intrauterine device: unusual pitfall. Clin Nucl Med 2007;32(2):128–9.

43. Sivin I, Batar I. State-of-the-art of non-hormonal methods of contraception: III. Intrauterine devices. Eur J Contracept Reprod Health Care 2010;15(2):96–112.

44. Romer W, Avril N, Dose J, et al. Metabolic characterization of ovarian tumors with positron-emission tomography and F-18 fluorodeoxyglucose. Rofo 1997;166(1):62–8 [in German].

45. Fenchel S, Grab D, Nuessle K, et al. Asymptomatic adnexal masses: correlation of FDG PET and histopathologic findings. Radiology 2002;223(3):780–8.

46. Kitajima K, Ueno Y, Maeda T, et al. Spectrum of fluorodeoxyglucose-positron emission tomography/computed tomography and magnetic resonance imaging findings of ovarian tumors. Jpn J Radiol 2011;29(9):605–8.

47. Toriihara A, Taniguchi Y, Negi M, et al. FDG PET/CT of a benign ovarian Brenner tumor. Clin Imaging 2012;36(5):650–3.

48. Tanaka YO, Okada S, Yagi T, et al. MRI of endometriotic cysts in association with ovarian carcinoma. AJR Am J Roentgenol 2010;194(2):355–61.

49. Jeffry L, Kerrou K, Camatte S, et al. Endometriosis with FDG uptake on PET. Eur J Obstet Gynecol Reprod Biol 2004;117(2):236–9.

50. Fastrez M, Nogarede C, Tondeur M, et al. Evaluation of 18FDG PET-CT in the diagnosis of endometriosis: a prospective study. Reprod Sci 2011;18(6):540–4.

Normal Variations and Benign Findings in Pediatric 18F-FDG-PET/CT

Frederick D. Grant, MD[a,b,*]

KEYWORDS

- 18F-FDG PET • PET/CT • Pediatric nuclear medicine • Pediatric imaging

KEY POINTS

- Infants and children provide special challenges to acquiring a technically adequate and diagnostically satisfactory positron emission tomography (PET) or PET/CT scan.
- Adequate prestudy preparation of patients and families is critical, and imaging protocols must pay particular attention to the pediatric spectrum of disease, the developmental needs of pediatric patients, and the goal of minimizing radiation exposure.
- Interpretation of pediatric PET with fludeoxyglucose F 18 (18F-FDG PET) and PET/CT requires knowledge of pediatric diseases and an appreciation for the patterns of tracer biodistribution that can be seen in infants and children.
- Protocols and departmental procedures must balance the developmental needs of children with the goal of acquiring a diagnostic imaging study that answers the clinical question.
- Achieving these goals can be facilitated by trained professional staff, including nuclear medicine physicians, nuclear medicine technologists, registered nurses, and child-life specialists, who have training and experience in pediatric imaging.

INTRODUCTION

The availability of PET, especially 18F-FDG PET/CT, has transformed pediatric nuclear medicine, especially pediatric nuclear oncology.[1–4] 18F-FDG PET and PET/CT have a wide variety of other indications,[1] including neurology,[5,6] sports medicine and orthopedics,[7] pediatric cardiology,[8] and infection imaging[9] in pediatric patients. Most PET and PET/CT studies use the glucose analog, 18F-FDG. The bone imaging agent [18F] sodium fluoride can be used to image both benign and malignant conditions of the skeleton,[7] but there is little pediatric experience with the few other PET radiopharmaceuticals approved for clinical use.[6,10]

Accurate interpretation of 18F-FDG PET and PET/CT requires a technically adequate study and knowledgeable interpretation of the resulting images. Pediatric 18F-FDG PET requires age-appropriate patient preparation, technically adequate acquisition, and appropriate image interpretation. Performing PET in pediatric patients requires consideration of the developmental stage of each patient and may require decisions about sedation and general anesthesia. A technically inadequate study can have decreased sensitivity for abnormal findings and may have technical artifacts that may obscure real findings. Accurate interpretation of the resulting images requires familiarity with the normal patterns of 18F-FDG distribution in children and the ability to recognize common developmental and physiologic patterns in the body (Fig. 1) and brain (Fig. 2).[11]

[a] Division of Nuclear Medicine and Molecular Imaging, Department of Radiology, Boston Children's Hospital, 300 Longwood Avenue, Boston, MA 02115, USA; [b] Joint Program in Nuclear Medicine, Harvard Medical School, 75 Francis Street, Boston, MA 02115, USA
* Division of Nuclear Medicine and Molecular Imaging, Boston Children's Hospital, 300 Longwood Avenue, Boston, MA 02115.
E-mail address: frederick.grant@childrens.harvard.edu

PET Clin 9 (2014) 195–208
http://dx.doi.org/10.1016/j.cpet.2013.12.002
1556-8598/14/$ – see front matter © 2014 Elsevier Inc. All rights reserved.

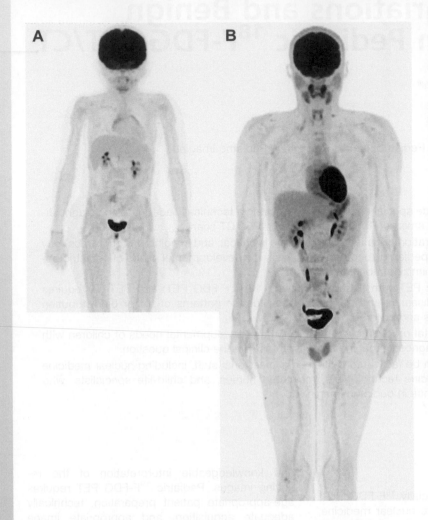

Fig. 1. Normal ^{18}F-FDG PET in pediatric patients. Maximum intensity projection images in (A) a 7-year-old girl and (B) a 17-year-old boy show typical patterns of normal physiologic uptake of ^{18}F-FDG. ^{18}F-FDG uptake is most intense in the brain. Other sites of normal physiologic uptake include the tonsils and liver. There is variable physiologic uptake in muscles, including skeletal muscle, myocardium, and the small muscles in the larynx and orbits. ^{18}F-FDG accumulation typically is seen in the renal collecting system, ureters, and bladder and may be seen in the gastrointestinal system. Physiologic uptake in the thymus is more common in younger pediatric patients than in teenagers or adults (A). Mild ^{18}F-FDG uptake can be seen in the growth centers of the wrists of an immature skeleton (A).

PATIENT PREPARATION FOR PEDIATRIC ^{18}F-FDG PET AND ^{18}F-FDG PET/CT

A technically adequate and diagnostically satisfactory ^{18}F-FDG PET or PET/CT depends on adequate patient preparation.[12–14] For pediatric patients, this requires that patients and families be involved in the preparation process. Although this might be accomplished with a mailing or on a departmental Web site, individual telephone contact made by a health care professional, such as a registered nurse or nuclear medicine technologist, before the study ensures the greatest likelihood of adequate patient preparation. A knowledgeable health care professional can provide individualized family education, address family concerns, identify potential problems that may affect the study, and assess the developmental needs of patients. Even patients and families with prior experience can benefit from a quick review of the patient preparation process.

For most ^{18}F-FDG PET and PET/CT of the torso, typically for an oncological indication[12] or for evaluating infection or inflammation,[15] prestudy fasting is important. Although less important for brain imaging, most guidelines recommend prestudy fasting before ^{18}F-FDG PET of the brain.[13] Conversely, ^{18}F-FDG PET for myocardial imaging requires enhancement of ^{18}F-FDG uptake in the myocardium,[14] although this procedure rarely is performed in children. Caloric intake stimulates insulin secretion, which can increase uptake of ^{18}F-FDG in skeletal and myocardial muscle. Therefore, except for cardiac imaging, patients should be fasting for at least 4 hours before administration of FDG and must remain fasting during the 1-hour uptake period after tracer administration. Prestudy caloric restriction includes feeding by nasogastric tube or percutaneous feeding tube. Most patients can continue to drink water, but must avoid sweetened or caffeine-containing beverages.[12,13] Even

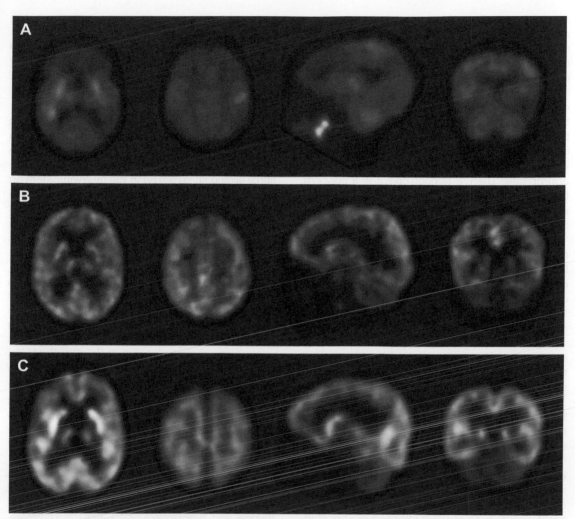

Fig. 2. Normal age-dependent patterns of ^{18}F-FDG uptake in the brain. In infants of 3 ages, ^{18}F-FDG PET images displayed in 2 transaxial, 1 saggital, and 1 coronal plane demonstrate increasing ^{18}F-FDG uptake and changing patterns of ^{18}F-FDG uptake that occur with brain maturation. (*A*) In a 2-month-old girl, cerebral uptake is highest in the sensorimotor cortex and cerebellum. (*B*) In a 9-month-old boy, there is increased ^{18}F-FDG uptake in the striatum and most of the cerebrum, but ^{18}F-FDG uptake remains relatively decreased in the frontal lobes. (*C*) In a 14-month-old boy, the pattern of ^{18}F-FDG uptake is similar to the adult pattern. In the cerebrum, ^{18}F-FDG uptake is greater in gray matter than in white matter, and uptake in the cerebellum is less than cerebral gray matter. The striatum also demonstrates intense uptake of ^{18}F-FDG. Increased uptake in the visual cortex reflects visual activity during the uptake period.

non-nutritional sweeteners may have a mild stimulatory effect on insulin secretion.[16] In patients receiving parenteral nutrition or hydration, all intravenous glucose sources must be discontinued for at least 4 hours before ^{18}F-FDG administration. If the study is performed with sedation or general anesthesia, however, patients must take nothing by mouth for the appropriate time before the procedure. If intravenous hydration is needed, it is important to confirm that all glucose-containing solutions, such as lactated Ringer solution, have been discontinued.

Adequate fasting can be a challenge in infants and young children. Most successful approaches coordinate the imaging study with a child's eating and sleeping schedule. Caloric intake after the 1-hour uptake period may have little effect on ^{18}F-FDG PET quality. Therefore, in older children, patient cooperation and successful completion of the scan may be improved by allowing a small snack after the uptake period and just before the start of imaging. Patients at increased risk of hypoglycemia, including infants, require special attention during prolonged fasting. Caloric intake still must be restricted before tracer administration and during the ^{18}F-FDG uptake period. If hypoglycemia is a clinical concern, infants can be breastfed after the 1-hour ^{18}F-FDG uptake period uptake, with hope that they may then sleep through the study. Patients in this age group, however, frequently require sedation or general anesthesia, for which patients must have nothing by mouth before the study. Depending on the requirements for anesthesia, intravenous hydration with a non–glucose-containing solution may be appropriate. Then, if hypoglycemia is a concern, blood glucose levels can be maintained with a dextrose-containing intravenous solution started after the 1-hour uptake period.

Hyperglycemia also can interfere with the quality of an ^{18}F-FDG PET or PET/CT. In patients with a high blood glucose level, circulating glucose can compete with cellular uptake of ^{18}F-FDG and decrease ^{18}F-FDG uptake in tissues of interest. This may be of greatest concern when imaging for oncological indications and of less concern when ^{18}F-FDG PET is performed to evaluate infection or inflammation.[15] Blood glucose should be checked, typically using a glucometer to test a finger-stick sample of capillary blood, before administration of ^{18}F-FDG. If the blood glucose level is greater than 200 mg/dL, then most guidelines recommend delaying the ^{18}F-FDG PET.[12,13] Some patients with diabetes mellitus arrive to their scheduled ^{18}F-FDG PET with marked hyperglycemia due to either poorly controlled diabetes or unrecognized nocturnal hyperglycemia. Even patients without a diagnosis of diabetes mellitus may develop hyperglycemia, such as when stressed or after starting glucocorticoid therapy. If at all possible, an ^{18}F-FDG PET or PET/CT study should be delayed until patients have better glycemic control.

Patients with diabetes mellitus require extra attention before an ^{18}F-FDG PET study. During fasting, insulin administration can produce hypoglycemia as well as stimulate nonspecific uptake of ^{18}F-FDG in muscle. If the diabetes mellitus is treated inadequately, however, then hyperglycemia can compete with tissue uptake of ^{18}F-FDG. Either of these can decrease the quality and impair the diagnostic accuracy of an ^{18}F-FDG PET. Any decision to alter the medical or nutritional regimen of a patient with diabetes mellitus should involve the patient's endocrinologist or primary care physician. These clinicians may not, however, be familiar with the techniques of ^{18}F-FDG PET and may depend on the expertise of a nuclear medicine physician for help in developing a plan for preparing a patient with diabetes mellitus.

Appropriate preparation of a patient with diabetes mellitus depends on whether the patient has type 1 (insulin-dependent) or type 2 (insulin-resistant) diabetes mellitus. Usually, scheduling the ^{18}F-FDG PET for early morning works best for patients with diabetes mellitus. Patients with type 1 diabetes mellitus must maintain appropriate basal blood insulin levels while fasting. Either subcutaneous injection of a long-acting insulin (typically at bedtime the prior evening) or subcutaneous infusion of insulin at a basal rate from an insulin pump can be used to produce adequate basal insulin levels. Patients, however, must not take additional sliding scale insulin in the morning before an ^{18}F-FDG PET study. Bolus insulin administration during fasting can result in fasting hypoglycemia and also will likely increase nonspecific muscle uptake of ^{18}F-FDG. If patients with diabetes mellitus present with fasting hyperglycemia, this may indicate a need for adjustment of the basal insulin dose.

Type 2 diabetes mellitus has been more common in adults than in children, but increasing numbers of children are developing this disease. Type 2 diabetes is the result of insulin resistance and is treated with dietary management, oral medications, or insulin administration. Most patients with type 2 diabetes mellitus do not develop marked hyperglycemia if they delay taking morning diabetes medications or insulin until after completion of an early morning ^{18}F-FDG PET or PET/CT. These patients should clearly understand if they are to take any oral diabetes medications while fasting, because some of these medications can result in fasting hypoglycemia. Use of metformin has been associated with intense ^{18}F-FDG uptake in the colon and in the small intestine.[17] Metformin also can increase skeletal muscle and liver uptake of ^{18}F-FDG.[18] Therefore, ideally, metformin should be discontinued 2 to 3 days before an ^{18}F-FDG PET study.[19]

Brown adipose tissue can be seen in as many as a third of all children having an ^{18}F-FDG PET or PET/CT study (**Fig. 3**). The prevalence of ^{18}F-FDG uptake may show seasonal variation but can be seen in any season. ^{18}F-FDG uptake in brown adipose tissue may be decreased with a variety of maneuvers. In the author's department, the incidence of significant uptake in brown adipose tissue was decreased from 33% to 9% by heating patients in a warm room (24 C) for at least 30 minutes before ^{18}F-FDG administration and then during the 60-minute uptake period.[20] Pharmacologic interventions to decrease ^{18}F-FDG uptake in brown adipose tissue have included a low dose of a β-blocker, such as propanolol[21]; a low dose of a benzodiazepine, such as diazepam[22]; or intravenous administration of fentanyl.[23] Brown adipose uptake also may be decreased by dietary restriction to a high-fat diet[24] for at least 12 hours before the study. One advantage of using patien

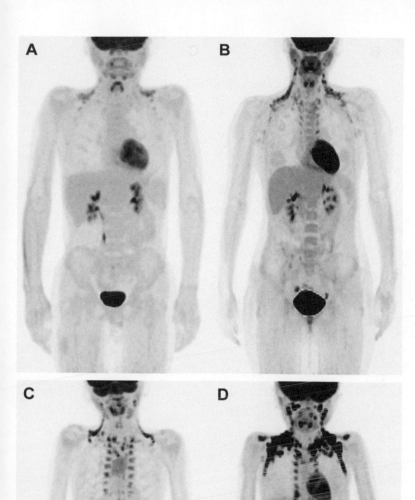

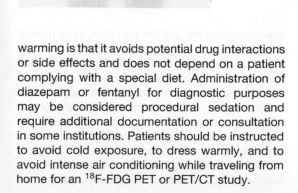

Fig. 3. ¹⁸F-FDG uptake in brown adipose tissue is common in children and adolescents. Many pediatric patients may have a mild brown adipose uptake in the neck or supraclavicular regions (*A*). Other patients (*B, C*) may have greater uptake that can include uptake in paraspinal brown adipose tissue. Occasionally, extensive uptake (*D*) may include pericardiac and perirenal brown adipose tissue. ¹⁸F-FDG uptake in brown adipose tissue can obscure sites of pathologic ¹⁸F-FDG uptake and decrease confidence in study interpretation. A variety of strategies have been used to decrease ¹⁸F-FDG uptake in brown adipose tissue. Note the marked variability in myocardial uptake despite similar prescan preparation.

warming is that it avoids potential drug interactions or side effects and does not depend on a patient complying with a special diet. Administration of diazepam or fentanyl for diagnostic purposes may be considered procedural sedation and require additional documentation or consultation in some institutions. Patients should be instructed to avoid cold exposure, to dress warmly, and to avoid intense air conditioning while traveling from home for an ¹⁸F-FDG PET or PET/CT study.

FDG uptake in muscle can be increased by intense or repetitive muscle use prior to ¹⁸F-FDG PET (**Fig. 4**). Widespread muscle uptake of ¹⁸F-FDG may decrease ¹⁸F-FDG available for uptake in tissues of interest, while either widespread or focal muscle uptake can obscure sites of pathologic uptake. Either of these can decrease the sensitivity of the ¹⁸F-FDG PET/CT study. Therefore, patients should avoid heavy physical exertion for at least 24 hours, and preferably 48 hours,

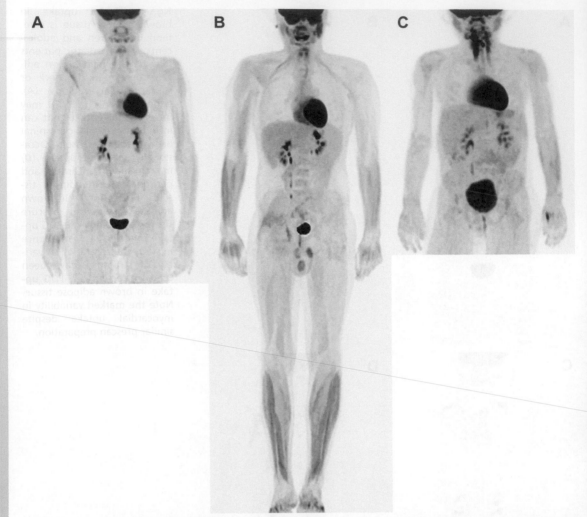

Fig. 4. Activity-related ^{18}F-FDG uptake in skeletal muscle. Nonpathologic muscle uptake can occur as the result of muscle use before or during the uptake period. (*A*) In a 17-year-old girl with neurofibromatosis of the scalp, increased uptake in the interosseous muscles of the right hand, muscles of the forearm, and right pectoral muscle reflects use of an electronic entertainment device during the uptake period. (*B*) In a 17-year-old male athlete treated for Ewing sarcoma, there is diffusely increased uptake throughout the skeletal muscles but most intense in the lower legs and forearms, after extreme physical exertion 1 day before ^{18}F-FDG PET/CT was performed. (*C, D*) In a 7-year-old boy treated for Burkitt lymphoma, intense uptake in the paraspinal muscles of the neck and upper back was attributed to patient posture during the uptake period. Muscle uptake in the left thumb also reflected electronic device use. (*E*) In a 2-year-old girl with Langerhans cell histiocytosis, there is extensive ^{18}F-FDG uptake in the muscles of respiration, including diaphragm, intercostal muscles, and sternocleidomastoid muscles, after prolonged crying during the uptake period.

before an ^{18}F-FDG PET or PET/CT. During the uptake period, both repetitive muscle activity, such as talking or chewing, and maintaining a static posture can increase FDG uptake in the involved muscles. In young children, increased muscle uptake of ^{18}F-FDG can occur after prolonged sucking or crying during the uptake period.[25]

After administration of ^{18}F-FDG, patients should stay in a quiet and warm environment during the uptake period. Patients may want to use electronic devices, including cell phones, electronic games, or laptop computers, but the repetitive hand motion required to operate these devices can increase ^{18}F-FDG uptake in the involved muscles. Quiet reading or movie watching can be appropriate activities, but patients should be reminded to avoid maintaining a single posture, because prolonged static contraction of neck or back muscles can increase ^{18}F-FDG uptake in the involved muscles (see **Fig. 4**). The preparations for brain ^{18}F-FDG PET of the brain (see **Fig. 2**) should limit sensory and emotional stimulation.[13] Patients should stay

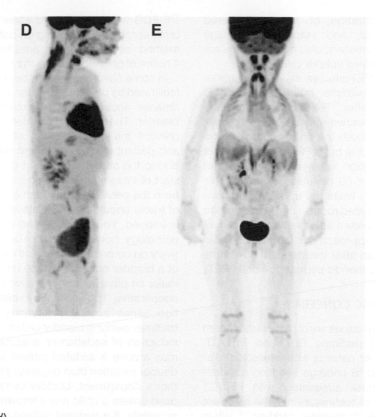

D   E

Fig. 4. (continued)

in a quiet, dimly lit room; should have limited interaction with others; and should not talk, speak, or read for a half-hour before FDG administration and during the uptake period. These limitations may not be practical, however, with every pediatric patient. Interaction with parents/caregivers, quiet reading, or use of electronic devices may be allowed or even necessary to maintain patient comfort or to gain patient cooperation. Determining the appropriate setting for the uptake period can be guided by the indications for the study and the region of interest within the brain. When imaging children and teenagers, flexibility is necessary to achieve a balance between acquiring the ideal imaging study and provoking an adverse behavioral response to conditions that are perceived as frightening or overly restrictive.

PET ACQUISITION

The radiopharmaceutical, camera geometry, clinical indication, and anatomic region to be imaged all influence the acquisition procedures for pediatric PET and PET/CT. The imaging protocols must be optimized for the equipment available for the study. Some PET cameras have septa, which allow images to be acquired in 2-D mode. If the septa are retracted or not available (as on most

cameras), then images are acquired in 3-D mode.[13] Time-of-flight circuitry also can influence acquisition parameters. ^{18}F-FDG PET in 2-D mode may require 4 to 6 minutes per bed position, whereas acquiring images in 3-D mode may require only 1.5 to 3 minutes per bed position. The size of the child and the length of the ring detector determine the number of bed positions needed to complete a study. Typically, no more than 2 bed positions and sometimes only 1 bed position is needed for brain PET/CT.

The radiopharmaceutical and the clinical indication for the PET study determine the uptake period, which is the time between radiopharmaceutical administration and the start of imaging. For oncological indications or for imaging infection or inflammation, ^{18}F-FDG PET of the torso (base of skull to thighs) or whole body (top of skull to feet) typically is started after a 60-minute uptake period. It is critical that the uptake period be consistent (less than 5 minutes of variation) if standard uptake values are compared from one study to the next.[25] Using a longer uptake period or acquiring a second ^{18}F-FDG PET has been suggested as an alternative approach to characterizing tumors,[26] but these methods have not entered routine clinical practice. Technical factors, including improper calibration of the dose calibrator or PET camera, subcutaneous infiltration of the administered radiopharmaceutical, and inappropriate image reconstruction parameters, also may affect the accuracy of the standard uptake value.[25]

Other ^{18}F-FDG PET studies may use a shorter uptake time. For example, brain PET usually is started 30 minutes after ^{18}F-FDG administration.[13] Two different approaches may be used when patients need PET of both the brain and body. One approach is to start the brain PET 30 minutes after ^{18}F-FDG administration followed by acquisition of the torso scan after 60 minutes of uptake. This approach, however, limits the uptake time that a patient stays in a heated room, if that is the method used to decrease brown adipose tissue uptake of ^{18}F-FDG. Another approach is to perform the torso or whole-body scan after the standard 60-minute uptake period and then to perform the brain PET.

SPECIAL PEDIATRIC CONCERNS

Some management issues are of particular concern when performing pediatric PET and PET/CT. Younger patients or patients with intellectual disabilities may need to undergo sedation or anesthesia to cooperate adequately with PET/CT imaging. Distraction techniques may be sufficient to complete a study in older children.[14] When used for brain ^{18}F-FDG PET, sedation or anesthesia should be administered as late as possible after

^{18}F-FDG administration to allow for unperturbed brain uptake.[13] Depending on patient age and the method of sedation or anesthesia, more than 4 hours of prestudy fasting may be required.

In some children, imaging pelvic disease may be facilitated by placing a bladder catheter, which decreases accumulation of excreted tracer in the bladder. The use of a bladder catheter also can prevent the contamination of the scanner bed and patient if a young patient inadvertently voids during the study. If a patient can void before the start of imaging and if torso imaging is performed from the pelvis to head, then only a small amount of tracer should be in the bladder when the pelvis is imaged. Young infants and children with pelvic pathology, however, may not be able to void effectively on command. On the other hand, placement of a bladder catheter can be unpleasant and may make an otherwise cooperative child become uncooperative. The approach to bladder catheterization varies among institutions. Some facilities routinely perform bladder catheterization only after induction of sedation or anesthesia,[14,27] but this may arouse a sedated patient and can required deeper sedation than originally planned. In the author's department, bladder catheterization is not used unless a child has a known voiding disorder or, rarely, if a sedated patient is found to have a large, filled bladder after the start of imaging (**Fig. 5**A).

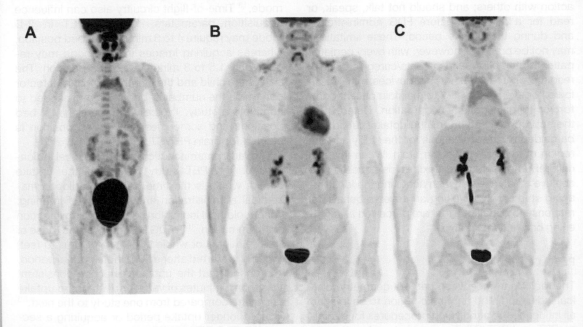

Fig. 5. Benign thymic uptake of ^{18}F-FDG. (*A*) In a 3-year-old girl, moderate uptake in a prominent thymus is typical for a child this age. (*B*) In a 14-year-old boy at the end of treatment of Hodgkin lymphoma, there is no ^{18}F-FDG uptake in the thymus, which can be typical for patients this age. (*C*) Six months after completion of treatment, moderate diffuse uptake demonstrates the thymic rebound phenomenon. Note the marked variability in myocardial uptake (*B, C*), despite similar prescan preparation.

The possibility of pregnancy must be considered in postpubertal girls and young women, and most institutions have standard policies guiding the determination of pregnancy status. At a minimum, postpubertal girls and young women should be asked if they might be pregnant. If a patient expresses concern about a possible pregnancy, a pregnancy test should be obtained before performing a PET or PET/CT scan. Depending on institutional policies and local governmental regulations, this may raise issues about patient confidentiality, parental or partner involvement, and the risks and benefits of the scheduled study. These discussions may necessitate involvement of the ordering clinician or primary care provider. More commonly in a pediatric practice, a patient's mother or other caregiver may be pregnant, which may require arrangements for other family members to accompany the patient during the PET or PET/CT study.[28]

IMAGE COREGISTRATION

The diagnostic accuracy of ¹⁸F-FDG PET can be improved by coregistration with anatomic imaging studies (CT, MR) or prior PET studies. Because all commercially available PET scanners are now integrated devices with both PET and CT capabilities, PET/CT fusion images can be obtained with little image manipulation. Coregistration with a previously acquired PET, diagnostic CT, or MR imaging using fusion software can be diagnostically useful. Software coregistration also is becoming more common in radiation therapy planning.[29] When brain ¹⁸F-FDG PET is used to evaluate a seizure disorder or brain tumor, correlative MR studies almost always are available and can be used to produce PET/MR fusion images.[6] Musculoskeletal tumors or intra-abdominal tumors may be imaged by MR imaging rather than CT, and PET/MR software coregistration can be useful for interpreting ¹⁸F-FDG PET studies. Recently introduced hybrid PET/MR imaging scanners may be well suited to pediatric applications,[30] but these have limited availability, and software coregistration of PET and MR imaging may provide a satisfactory approach to improving diagnostic certainty while decreasing radiation dose.

PET/CT

A CT acquired as part of a PET/CT study can serve as a stand-alone diagnostic study (with or without intravenous contrast, as indicated), as a nondiagnostic study for anatomic correlation, or for attenuation correction only.[12] CT energy settings are determined by the intended use and patient size. Depending on patient size, an attenuation-only CT can be acquired with an energy of only 16 to 30 mA.[31] A CT scan used for attenuation correction should be acquired with the same patient positioning and with the same breathing pattern as the ¹⁸F-FDG PET.[12] For example, the chest should be imaged during tidal breathing or with a midbreath breath hold. If this is not done, misregistration of the attenuation map and PET can create attenuation artifacts that may decrease the diagnostic accuracy of the ¹⁸F-FDG PET.

The appropriate use of intravenous and oral contrast for pediatric ¹⁸F-FDG PET/CT has not been resolved.[12,25] The use of either contrast agent implies that the CT is a diagnostic-quality CT scan, which will require a higher radiation dose than a CT intended for attenuation correction or localization. If a recent diagnostic CT has been performed, then performing another one as part of the PET/CT may not be necessary. Alternatively, if a diagnostic CT could be acquired as part of the PET/CT, then a separate diagnostic CT might be avoided, which can lessen the overall radiation dose to a patient. The use of an oral contrast agent raises the possibility of attenuation artifacts that might result from minor misregistration between the CT and PET acquisitions. This risk may be greatest with barium-containing oral contrast agents. The risk of artifacts may be lower with negative contrast agents, such as water and with iodinated oral contrast, possibly because iodinated contrast agents typically are used in diluted form and have a lower density than barium contrast agents. Oral contrast agents should be given only with noncaloric, nonsweetened liquids if they are administered before the ¹⁸F-FDG PET scan. Similarly, if a CT acquired early during intravenous contrast injection is used for attenuation correction of the PET, attenuation artifacts can occur around vessels containing a transiently high concentration of iodinated contrast.

Developing the CT and PET imaging protocols for ¹⁸F-FDG PET/CT must be customized for the medical and developmental needs of each patient. In the absence of a specific clinical indication, the routine acquisition of high-energy diagnostic CT throughout the PET field of view is inappropriate in pediatric patients. For each patient, the PET and CT imaging protocols should be guided by clinical indication, sites of known disease, and the information that can be provided by each study, while guided by the principles of as low as reasonably achievable (ALARA).[32]

NORMAL PATTERNS OF ^{18}F-FDG UPTAKE IN PEDIATRICS

In pediatric nuclear medicine, familiarity with the normal patterns of ^{18}F-FDG distribution in children is needed for an accurate interpretation of an ^{18}F-FDG PET or PET/CT study. For example, pathologic uptake must be distinguished from the normal patterns of physiologic uptake and excretion of ^{18}F-FDG.[33-35] In addition, typical physiologic uptake may obscure nearby abnormal uptake.

The normal brain is characterized by a high level of ^{18}F-FDG uptake. In adults and older children, up to 6% of an administered dose of ^{18}F-FDG may be taken up in the brain,[36] which reflects the high dependence of the brain on glucose for energy. Glucose provides approximately 95% of the energy used by the brain.[13] In infants, however, glucose uptake is less robust and patterns of glucose uptake differ from older children (see Fig. 2).[11] In older children, ^{18}F-FDG uptake is most intense uptake in the gray matter and basal ganglia (see Fig. 2), and neuronal activation increases ^{18}F-FDG uptake. For example, increased ^{18}F-FDG uptake can be seen in the visual cortex after visual activation. Therefore, patients ideally remain in a dim, quiet room with little sensory or emotional stimulation during the uptake period before a brain ^{18}F-FDG PET. The normal pattern of intense ^{18}F-FDG uptake limits the use of ^{18}F-FDG PET for evaluation of brain tumors because it may be difficult to discriminate tumor uptake from normal brain uptake. Pathologic uptake in the adjacent scalp or skull base also can be obscured by intense uptake in the adjacent brain.

FDG uptake in lymphatic tissue can depend on location of the lymphatic tissue, age of the patient, and concomitant conditions that may stimulate lymphatic uptake. Normal physiologic ^{18}F-FDG uptake is seen in lymphatic tissue in the Waldeyer ring, including the palatine tonsils and adenoids (see Figs. 1, 4, and 5). Children typically have prominent uptake in these tissues, but this is a nonspecific finding. Normal physiologic uptake can obscure disease, whereas increased uptake in response to an upper respiratory infection can be difficult to distinguish from a more severe disease. As a general rule, physiologic ^{18}F-FDG uptake in the tonsils is more likely symmetrical, whereas more serious disease, such as lymphoma, may be asymmetrical.[37]

Other sites of normal uptake in the head and neck include mild, and usually symmetric, ^{18}F-FDG uptake in salivary glands and pharyngeal muscles. Uptake in the tongue or muscles of mastication can be seen after vigorous or repetitive chewing, for example, in patients who chew gum during the uptake period. In infants, suckling can increase ^{18}F-FDG uptake in oral muscles. Laryngeal uptake can range from mild to intense, reflecting recent talking or crying. As in adults, asymmetric laryngeal uptake is more concerning for pathology, because it may suggest either local involvement by FDG-avid disease or unilateral vocal cord paralysis.

Children can demonstrate variable ^{18}F-FDG uptake in the heart, and intense myocardial uptake can occur even after well-documented standard fasting (see Figs. 3 and 5). In adults, other dietary interventions, such as a high-fat, low-carbohydrate diet, have been used to decrease myocardial uptake before torso or whole-body ^{18}F-FDG PET/CT.[24] This might be useful in patients with FDG-avid disease located near the heart, but there has been little reported experience using these diets in children.

The organs of hematopoiesis and the immune system, including the thymus, bone marrow, and spleen, have patterns of ^{18}F-FDG uptake that can help distinguish normal physiologic uptake from pathologic uptake. In the thymus, diffuse ^{18}F-FDG uptake rarely indicates disease in children (see Fig. 5). A diffuse pattern of uptake usually represents age-related physiologic activation. A similar pattern, termed thymic rebound, can be observed 4 to 6 months after completion of chemotherapy.[38] The inverse-V pattern of uptake is typical of the thymus, but correlation or coregistration with a chest CT can be used to confirm that the uptake is in the thymus. Diffuse bone marrow uptake of ^{18}F-FDG is a well-described response to cancer therapy, including physiologic rebound after chemotherapy and pharmacologic stimulation with colony-stimulating factors used to hasten marrow recovery (Fig. 6).[33,39] Occasionally, diffuse marrow uptake of ^{18}F-FDG can represent incidental non–treatment-related marrow stimulation, such as the response to anemia or a systemic inflammatory process.[33] In some patients presenting with Hodgkin disease, diffuse ^{18}F-FDG uptake may be seen in bone marrow, but this rarely represents disease and likely reflects cytokine-mediated marrow stimulation. Alternatively, in pediatric cancer patients, focal ^{18}F-FDG uptake in bone marrow rarely reflects treatment-related marrow stimulation and usually represents marrow involvement by disease. After treatment of marrow infiltrating disease, follow-up ^{18}F-FDG PET may show regions of minimal ^{18}F-FDG uptake at sites of former bone marrow disease. In the same way, minimal marrow uptake may be seen within the field of therapeutic radiation. These patterns may be most apparent when normal marrow exhibits robust ^{18}F-FDG uptake related to treatment-related marrow stimulation.

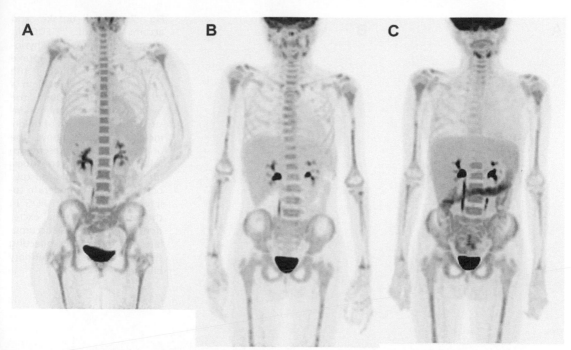

Fig. 6. Benign, malignancy-related ^{18}F-FDG uptake in bone marrow. In patients with lymphoma or a solid tumor, widespread diffuse marrow uptake rarely represents disease and more likely reflects physiologic or pharmacologic marrow stimulation. (*A*) In a 16-year-old girl successfully treated for Hodgkin disease, diffuse ^{18}F-FDG uptake in the expected locations of bone marrow likely represents treatment-related marrow stimulation. (*B*) In a 9-year-old girl treated for metastatic rhabdomyosarcoma, there is treatment-related marrow stimulation with absent or heterogenous uptake at many prior sites of metastatic osseous disease. (*C*) In the same patient, after radiation therapy to the upper torso, marrow uptake of ^{18}F-FDG is decreased in the upper spine and ribs, whereas marrow uptake is normalizing at prior sites of osseous metastases.

Normal physiologic distribution of ^{18}F-FDG can be seen at sites throughout the gastrointestinal tract.[34] Focal uptake at the gastroesophageal junction is a normal finding. Substantial diffuse or regional ^{18}F-FDG uptake along the esophagus more likely represents an inflammatory process. Most commonly this is seen in oncology patients, and esophageal uptake represents post-treatment mucositis related to either chemotherapy or radiation. Patients with other forms of esophagitis are rarely imaged with ^{18}F-FDG PET, but increased esophageal uptake of ^{18}F-FDG also can occur with chemical esophagitis related to gastroesophageal reflux, or, rarely, secondary to caustic ingestion.

In the stomach, ^{18}F-FDG uptake in the gastric wall can be physiological but also may indicate a pathological neoplastic or inflammatory process. Correlation with CT sometimes is of benefit but, if clinically important, tissue biopsy may be necessary to determine if gastric ^{18}F-FDG uptake reflects underlying pathology. In the small and large intestines, the pattern of ^{18}F-FDG uptake may help distinguish physiologic from pathologic uptake.[40,41] Typical physiologic ^{18}F-FDG uptake

can be multifocal and widespread. The mechanism of this uptake remains unclear. Physiologic intestinal uptake might be in mucosa, muscle, or luminal contents. Regional, segmental, or widespread diffuse intestinal ^{18}F-FDG uptake more likely represents an inflammatory process.[35] For example, terminal ileitis may come to attention due to incidental ^{18}F-FDG uptake identified on an ^{18}F-FDG PET/CT. A single intense focus of ^{18}F-FDG uptake is worrisome for disease and, in particular, raises concern for neoplasm.[36]

^{18}F-FDG is excreted through the urinary system, so tracer accumulation commonly is seen in the kidneys, renal collecting systems, ureters, and bladder (**Fig. 7**).[34,42] Tracer accumulation in ureters usually can be identified by the distinctive contours of the ureters and by correlation with CT. This may be particularly helpful if there is focal urinary tracer accumulation within the urinary collecting system. ^{18}F-FDG accumulation in the collecting system can be minimized by encouraging patient hydration. Although routine use of pharmacologic diuresis has been advocated in the past, diuretics are rarely, if ever, used for imaging children.[35] Bladder catheterization may be helpful in

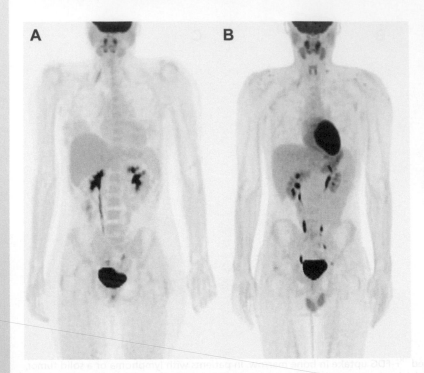

Fig. 7. Normal uptake and accumulation of ^{18}F-FDG in the genitourinary tract. Physiologic ^{18}F-FDG uptake frequently is identified in the reproductive organs. (A) In a 15-year-old girl around the ovulation phase of her menstrual cycle, 2 regions of mildly increased uptake above the urinary bladder represent uptake in the fallopian tubes. (B) Peripubertal and postpubertal boys have moderate-to-intense uptake of ^{18}F-FDG in the testes. Due to renal excretion, ^{18}F-FDG typically accumulates in the renal collecting systems, ureters, and urinary bladder.

selected circumstances, such as in a sedated patient in whom tracer accumulation within the bladder may obscure ^{18}F-FDG uptake in nearby disease. Rarely, collecting system obstruction or hydronephrosis is identified on ^{18}F-FDG PET or PET/CT. Tracer accumulation in congenital variants, such as a dilated renal calyx, an ectopic or horseshoe kidney, or a bladder diverticulum, must be recognized to avoid misinterpreting these findings as a site of FDG-avid disease.[43] Persistent ^{18}F-FDG uptake in the renal cortex is abnormal and has a broad differential, including infection, leukemia, and lymphoma.[44]

Uptake of ^{18}F-FDG in the reproductive organs varies with pubertal status and, in female patients, with the menstrual cycle.[45–47] In male patients, physiologic uptake of ^{18}F-FDG can be seen in testes,[45] especially in peripubertal and postpubertal young men (see **Fig. 7**). In premenarcheal female patients, ^{18}F-FDG uptake should not be seen in these organs. After menarche, ^{18}F-FDG uptake in the ovaries and fallopian tubes can be seen during follicular genesis and ovulation, at the midcycle.[46,47] Fallopian tube uptake, if present, is typically bilateral (see **Fig. 7**), whereas ovarian uptake is generally unilateral.[46] Endometrial uptake seems most intense during the menstruation but also may be increased in the ovulatory phase of the menstrual cycle.[47] Therefore, it is necessary to know the pubertal status and menstrual phase to adequately interpret these findings in female patients.

Increased muscle uptake of ^{18}F-FDG can decrease uptake in sites of pathology and may require the imaging study to be repeated.[48] In muscle, increased ^{18}F-FDG uptake can be seen for up to 2 days after heavy or repetitive muscle exertion (see **Fig. 4**), with the pattern of muscle uptake reflecting the involved muscles. Diffusely increased muscle uptake is seen if patients have not fasted before administration of ^{18}F-FDG. Less commonly, widespread ^{18}F-FDG uptake in muscle reflects an inflammatory myositis or rhabdomyolysis. Patients with hyperthyroidism can have diffusely increased uptake in muscles and decreased hepatic uptake.[49] Compensatory muscle activity, such as increased muscle uptake in leg muscles after disuse or after amputation of the contralateral limb, can lead to increased muscle uptake of ^{18}F-FDG. In the same patients, use of a cane or crutches can increase ^{18}F-FDG uptake in arm and shoulder muscles. An increased work of breathing related to respiratory distress or even crying can lead to increased ^{18}F-FDG uptake in the diaphragm, intercostal muscles, and accessory muscles of respiration (see **Fig. 4**E).

Skeletal uptake of ^{18}F-FDG is a nonspecific finding that may represent pathology or normal physiology. In children, physiologic uptake of ^{18}F-FDG can be seen as sites of bone growth, such as the physes of the long bones (see **Fig. 1**A). Increased ^{18}F-FDG uptake also has been reported in growth arrest lines (Harris lines) that can occur after resolution of skeletal growth arrest related to illness, starvation, or prolonged immobilization.[50]

SUMMARY

Infants and children provide special challenges to acquiring a technically adequate and diagnostically satisfactory PET or PET/CT scan. Adequate prestudy preparation of patients and families is critical. Imaging protocols must pay particular attention to the pediatric spectrum of disease, the developmental needs of pediatric patients, and the goal of minimizing radiation exposure. Interpretation of pediatric ^{18}F-FDG PET and PET/CT requires knowledge of pediatric diseases and an appreciation for the patterns of tracer biodistribution that can be seen in infants and children. Issues, such as sedation or anesthesia, rarely a concern in adult nuclear medicine, are a normal part of routine pediatric PET and PET/CT. Protocols and departmental procedures must balance the developmental needs of children with the goal of acquiring a diagnostic imaging study that answers the clinical question. Achieving this goal can be facilitated by trained professional staff, including nuclear medicine physicians, nuclear medicine technologists, registered nurses, and child-life specialists, who have training and experience in pediatric imaging.

REFERENCES

1. Jadvar H, Connolly LP, Fahey FH, et al. PET and PET/CT in pediatric oncology. Semin Nucl Med 2007;37:316–31.
2. Grant FD, Dubach L, Treves ST. ^{18}F-fluorodeoxy-glucose PET and PET/CT in pediatric musculoskeletal malignancies. PET Clin 2010;5:349–61.
3. Portwine C, Marriot C, Barr RD. PET imaging for pediatric oncology: an assessment of the evidence. Pediatr Blood Cancer 2010;55:1048–61.
4. Grant FD, Treves ST. Nuclear medicine and molecular imaging of the pediatric chest: current practical imaging assessment. Radiol Clin North Am 2011;49:1025–51.
5. Patil S, Biassoni L, Borgwardt L. Nuclear medicine in pediatric neurology and neurosurgery: epilepsy and brain tumors. Semin Nucl Med 2007;37: 357–81.
6. Kim S, Salamon N, Jackson HA, et al. PET imaging in pediatric neuroradiology: current and future applications. Pediatr Radiol 2010;40:82–96.
7. Grant FD, Fahey FH, Packard AB, et al. Skeletal PET with ^{18}F-fluoride: applying new technology to an old tracer. J Nucl Med 2008;49:68–78.
8. Jadvar H, Alavi A, Mavi A, et al. PET in pediatric diseases. Radiol Clin North Am 2005;43:135–52.
9. Kaste SC. PET-CT in children: where is it appropriate? Pediatr Radiol 2011;41:S509–13.
10. Weckesser M. Molecular imaging with positron emission tomography in paediatric oncology–FDG and beyond. Pediatr Radiol 2009;39:S450–5.
11. Chugani HT, Phelops ME, Mazziotta JC. Positron emission tomography study of human brain functional development. Ann Neurol 1987;22: 487–97.
12. Dulbeke D, Coleman RE, Guiberteau MJ, et al. Procedure guideline for tumor imaging with ^{18}F-FDG PET/CT 1.0. J Nucl Med 2006;47:885–95.
13. Waxman AD, Herholz K, Lewis DH, et al. Society of Nuclear Medicine procedure guideline for FDG PET brain imaging. Available at: snmmi.files.cms-plus.com/docs/jnm30551_online.pdf. Accessed January 14, 2014.
14. McQuattie S. Pediatric PET/CT imaging: tips and techniques. J Nucl Med Technol 2008;36:171–8.
15. Rabkin Z, Israel O, Keidar Z. Do hyperglycemia and diabetes affect the incidence of false-negative ^{18}F-FDG PET/CT studies in patients evaluated for infection or inflammation and cancer? A comparative analysis. J Nucl Med 2010; 51:1015–20.
16. Liang Y, Steinbach G, Maier V, et al. The effect of artificial sweetener on insulin secretion. 1. The effect of acesulfame K on insulin secretion in the rat (studies in vivo). Horm Metab Res 1987;19: 233–8.
17. Gontier E, Fourme E, Wartski M, et al. High and typical ^{18}F-FDG bowel uptake in patients treated with metformin. Eur J Nucl Med Mol Imaging 2008;35:95–9.
18. Bybel B, Greenberg ID, Paterson J, et al. Increased F-18 FDG intestinal uptake in diabetic patients on metformin: a matched case-control analysis. Clin Nucl Med 2011;36:452–6.
19. Ozülker T, Ozülker F, Mert M, et al. Clearance of the high intestinal ^{18}F-FDG uptake associated with metformin after stopping the drug. Eur J Nucl Med Mol Imaging 2010;37:1011–7.
20. Zukotynski KA, Fahey FA, Laffin S, et al. Constant ambient temperature of 24°C significantly reduces FDG uptake by brown adipose tissue in children. Eur J Nucl Med Mol Imaging 2009;36:602–6.
21. Söderlund V, Larsson SA, Jacobsson H. Reduction of FDG uptake in brown adipose tissue in clinical patients by a single dose of propanolol. Eur J Nucl Med Mol Imaging 2007;34:1018–22.
22. Barrington SF, Maisey MN. Skeletal muscle uptake of fluorine-18-FDG: effect of oral diazepam. J Nucl Med 1996;37:1127–9.
23. Gelfand MJ, O'Hara SM, Curtwright LA, et al. Premedication to block [^{18}F]FDG uptake in the brown adipose tissue of pediatric and adolescent patients. Pediatr Radiol 2005;35:984–90.

24. Williams G, Kolodny GM. Method for decreasing uptake of ^{18}F-FDG by hypermetabolic brown adipose tissue on PET. Am J Roentgenol 2008;190:1406–9.

25. Boellaard R. Standards for PET image acquisition and quantitative data analysis. J Nucl Med 2009; 50:11S–20S.

26. Hustinx R, Smith RJ, Benard F, et al. Dual time point fluorine-18 fluorodeoxyglucose positron emission tomography: a potential method to differentiate malignancy from inflammation and normal tissue in the head and neck. Eur J Nucl Med 1999;26:1345–8.

27. Roberts EG, Shulkin BA. Technical issues in performed PET studies in pediatric patients. J Nucl Med Technol 2004;32:5–9.

28. McCarville MB. PET-CT imaging in pediatric oncology. Cancer Imaging 2009;9:35–43.

29. Scripes PG, Yaparpalvi R. Technical aspects of positron emission tomography/computed tomography in radiotherapy treatment planning. Semin Nucl Med 2012;42:283–8.

30. Antoch G, Bockisch A. Combined PET/MRI: a new dimension in whole-body oncology imaging? Eur J Nucl Med Mol Imaging 2009;36:S113–20.

31. Fahey FH. Dosimetry of pediatric PET/CT. J Nucl Med 2009;50:1483–91.

32. Chawla SC, Federman N, Zhang D, et al. Estimated cumulative radiation dose from PET/CT in children with malignancies: a 5-year retrospective review. Pediatr Radiol 2010;40:681–6.

33. Gordon BA, Flanagan FL, Dehdashti F. Whole-body positron emission tomography: normal variations, pitfalls, and technical considerations. Am J Roentgenol 1997;169:1675–80.

34. Shreve PD, Anzai Y, Wahl RL. Pitfalls in oncologic diagnosis with FDG PET imaging: physiologic and benign variants. Radiographics 1999;19:61–77.

35. Shammas A, Lim R, Charron M. Pediatric FDG PET/CT: physiological uptake, normal variants, and benign conditions. Radiographics 2009;29: 1467–86.

36. Ak I, Stokkel MP, Pauwels EK. Positron emission tomography with 2-[18F]fluoro-2-deoxy-D-glucose in oncology. II: the clinical value in detecting and staging primary tumours. J Cancer Res Clin Oncol 2000;126:560–74.

37. Sarji SA. Physiological uptake in FDG PET simulating disease. Biomed Imaging Interv J 2006;2:e59.

38. Brink I, Reinhardt MJ, Hoegerle S, et al. Increased metabolic activity in the thymus studied with FDG

PET: age dependency and frequency after chemotherapy. J Nucl Med 2001;42:591–5.

39. Yao WJ, Hoh CK, Hawkins RA, et al. Quantitative PET imaging of bone marrow glucose metabolic response to hematopoietic cytokines. J Nucl Med 1995;36:794–9.

40. Tatlidil R, Jadvar H, Bading JR, et al. Incidental colonic fluorodeoxyglucose uptake: correlation with colonoscopic and histopathological findings. Radiology 2002;224:783–7.

41. Cho SH, Kim SW, Kim WC, et al. Incidental focal colorectal ^{18}F-fluorodeoxyglucose uptake on positron emission tomography/computed tomography. World J Gastroenterol 2013;19:3453–8.

42. Vesselle HJ, Miraldi FD. FDG PET of the retroperitoneum: normal anatomy, variants, pathologic conditions, and strategies to avoid diagnostic pitfalls. Radiographics 1998;18:805–23.

43. Subhas N, Patel PV, Pannu HK, et al. Imaging of pelvic malignancies with in-line FDG PET-CT: case examples and common pitfalls of FDG PET. Radiographics 2005;25:1031–43.

44. Zukotynski K, Lewis A, O'Regan K, et al. PET/CT and renal pathology: a blind spot for radiologists? Part 2 – lymphoma, leukemia, and metastatic disease. Am J Roentgenol 2012;199:168–74.

45. Kitajima K, Nakamoto Y, Senda M, et al. Normal uptake of ^{18}F-FDG in the testis: an assessment by PET/CT. Ann Nucl Med 2007;21:405–10.

46. Yun M, Cho A, Lee JH, et al. Physiologic ^{18}F-FDG uptake in the fallopian tubes at mid cycle on PET/CT/. J Nucl Med 2010;51:682–5.

47. Lerman H, Metser U, Grisaru D, et al. Normal and abnormal ^{18}F-FDG endometrial and ovarian uptake in pre- and postmenopausal patients: assessment by PET/CT. J Nucl Med 2004;45:266–71.

48. Lindholm H, Johannsson O, Jonsson C, et al. The distribution of FDG at PET examinations constitutes a relative mechanism: significant effects at activity quantification in patients with a high muscle uptake. Eur J Nucl Med Mol Imaging 2012;39: 1685–90.

49. Chen YK, Chen YL, Tsui CC, et al. The significance of alteration in 2-[fluorine-18] fluoro-2-deoxy-d-glucose uptake in the liver and skeletal muscles of patients with hyperthyroidism. Acad Radiol 2013;20:1218–23.

50. Lim R, Carrasquillo JA. ^{18}F-FDG uptake in metaphyseal growth arrest lines: a case study. Clin Nucl Med 2012;37:993–4.

Differential Background Clearance of Fluorodeoxyglucose Activity in Normal Tissues and its Clinical Significance

Gang Cheng, MD, PhD[a,b,*], Abass Alavi[b], Nam Ju Lee, MD[b],
Scott R. Akers, MD, PhD[a]

KEYWORDS

- Fluorodeoxyglucose • PET • SUV • Distribution time • Background activity • Delayed imaging

KEY POINTS

- The clearance of 2-deoxy-2-[18F]fluoro-D-glucose (FDG) activity in normal tissues varies significantly with extended distribution time.
- Although most tissues have lower standardized uptake value (SUV) on 2-hour/3-hour delayed images, others may have stable or higher FDG activity with longer distribution times.
- The continuously decreased SUV on delayed imaging in some tissues, especially in the liver, indicates that longer distribution time will decrease background activity, increase lesion-to-background ratio, and thus improve imaging quality, whereas the continuously increased SUV from 1 to 3 hours in the heart suggest that longer distribution time will improve detection of viable myocardium in a viability study.

INTRODUCTION

The imaging modality of 2-deoxy-2-[18F]fluoro-D-glucose (FDG) PET/computed tomography (CT) has been studied intensively over the past 10 years, because it has evolved into a major form of clinical evaluation. The underlying mechanism of FDG-PET is the differential glycolytic activity in normal versus pathologic tissues. However, intracellular accumulation of FDG is not a specific finding for any pathologic condition, and the standardized uptake value (SUV) of FDG is not a fixed value for any tissues.

Tracer distribution time significantly affects tissue FDG activity on FDG-PET imaging. SUV obtained at an early time point may not be equivalent to the value obtained at a later time point. This possibility limits the direct comparison of two studies performed with different distribution times, and it also has to be considered when using the uptake of the mediastinal/aortic blood pool or the hepatic activity as an internal reference,[1,2]

This study was supported in part by a pilot grant from the Department of Veterans Affairs (VISN 4 CPPF Grant). The content of this article does not necessarily reflect the views of the US Department of Veterans Affairs or of the US Government.

Conflict of interest: None.

[a] Department of Radiology, Philadelphia VA Medical Center, 3900 Woodland Avenue, Philadelphia, PA 19104, USA; [b] Department of Radiology, Hospital of the University of Pennsylvania, 3400 Spruce Street, Philadelphia, PA 19104, USA

* Corresponding author. Department of Radiology, Philadelphia VA Medical Center, 3900 Woodland Avenue, Philadelphia, PA 19104.

E-mail address: gangcheng99@yahoo.com

PET Clin 9 (2014) 209–216
http://dx.doi.org/10.1016/j.cpet.2013.12.001
1556-8598/14/$ – see front matter Published by Elsevier Inc.

because FDG uptake in these reference tissues is similarly affected by tracer distribution time. In addition, delayed or dual-time-point FDG-PET imaging has been proposed in order to follow the uptake of the agent in a dynamic fashion and to enhance the diagnostic accuracy,[3,4] because delayed imaging has been reported to improve the differentiation between benign inflammation and malignancy.[5–8] Knowledge of dynamic FDG uptake in different tissues may help the nuclear medicine physician to decide when to request an additional delayed imaging (eg, an equivocal lesion in a tissue that normally clears background activity over time) or not to request such a delayed imaging.

This article analyzes the background activity clearance of the various tissues by quantifying the FDG uptake at 1 hour, 2 hours, and 3 hours after tracer injection on FDG-PET/CT to evaluate its clinical significance in each tissue type. This article was expanded from our prior study on this topic[9] as more patients were recruited and more data were accumulated.

SUBJECTS AND METHODS
Patients

Fifty nine patients (including 30 patients as previously reported[9]) with suspected lung cancer were prospectively recruited for our study of multiple time point FDG PET/CT scan. The study was approved by our institutional review board (IRB) at the Philadelphia Veterans' Affairs Medical Center. Informed consent was obtained from all 59 patients included in this analysis. All patients had overnight fasting. The blood sugar level was less than 200 mg/dL before the study.

Imaging

Whole-body FDG-PET/CT images were acquired from the skull base to midthighs, at 1 hour, 2 hours, and 3 hours after intravenous injection of 370 to 555 MBq (10–15 mCi) FDG using a dedicated PET/CT scanner (the Biograph 64 hybrid PET/CT imaging systems; Siemens Medical Solutions, Inc). Patients remained fasted until the end of the study and remained resting on a bed between the studies to minimize muscle uptake. A diluted oral contrast (MD-Gastroview, Mallinckrodt Inc) was given to every patient. No intravenous contrast was administered. The images were reconstructed in axial, coronal, and sagittal plans for interpretation.

Data Analysis

All FDG-PET/CT studies were reviewed by a nuclear medicine physician and a radiologist experienced in PET imaging. The maximum SUVs (SUV_{max}) were measured for semiquantitative analysis in patients meeting our criteria: (1) completion of serial whole-body ^{18}F-FDG-PET/CT images at 1 hour, 2 hours, and 3 hours after tracer injection; (2) absence of malignancy in the area of interest; (3) absence of artifacts in the area of interest. A large region of interest (ROI) was drawn to include the major part of an organ without including nearby tissues for the normal tissue activity. For the blood pool activity, the ROI was placed at the lower descending thoracic aorta without including the aortic wall. For the heart, the ROI was placed at the region of the highest FDG activity in the left ventricular (LV) lateral wall. For SUV quantitation, three-dimensional (3D) measurement was used for most tissues, whereas two-dimensional measurement was used for the lungs, liver, spleen, and prostate gland to avoid potential errors induced by inclusion of an unwanted uptake on 3D measurement, such as inflammatory changes in the lung or urine activity near the prostate gland.

For each organ or tissue, only 1 SUV_{max} was obtained for analysis, except for the following conditions: (1) for bone uptake, several sites were selected and SUV_{max} was obtained for each site; (2) for lymph nodes, SUV_{max} was obtained from the largest node in each side of nodes; (3) for brown fat activity, SUV_{max} was obtained from each area of discrete focal uptake.

The SUV_{max} values were analyzed using paired 1-way analysis of variance (ANOVA) test to determine the significance of differences for dynamic SUV values, using the GraphPad Prism 4 (GraphPad Software, Inc, San Diego, CA). Probability values less than .05 were considered significant. The retention index (RI)[5,8] is defined as the difference in SUV between early and delayed FDG-PET imaging as a percentage of the initial uptake (RI = ($SUV_{delayed}$ − SUV_{early})/SUV_{early} × 100%).[9]

RESULTS
Tissues with Decreased FDG Uptake on Delayed Images

The delayed FDG-PET imaging showed significantly decreased FDG activity in the blood pool of the aorta, the liver, spleen, lung, pancreas, adrenal gland, skeletal muscle, and lymph nodes. This decrease was observed in 48 of 49 patients for the liver and 46 of 50 patients for the aortic blood pool activity both from 1 to 2 hours and from 2 to 3 hours. However, the degree of the decrease in FDG activity was variable depending on tissue types. The continued decrease of SUV_{max} was more remarkable in the aortic blood pool and liver than in other tissues. There was significant decrease of the SUV$_{max}$ values in the aortic blood pool, liver, and spleen with longer distribution time, from 1 hour to 2 hours and also from 2 hours to 3 hours. In contrast, a smaller decrease of the SUV$_{max}$ was presented in the lungs, pancreas, adrenal gland, inguinal nodes, and skeletal muscles: these tissues had significant decrease of FDG activity from 1 hour to 2 hours and from 1 hour to

3 hours, but no significant difference from 2 hours to 3 hours (**Fig. 1**).

We observed that dynamics of ^{18}F-FDG uptake of the axillary lymph nodes were affected by the site of tracer injection. Consistent decrease in SUV$_{max}$ was observed in the inguinal or axillary lymph nodes on the side contralateral to the injection. However, the SUV$_{max}$ in the axillary nodes on the injection side did not decrease in activity on the

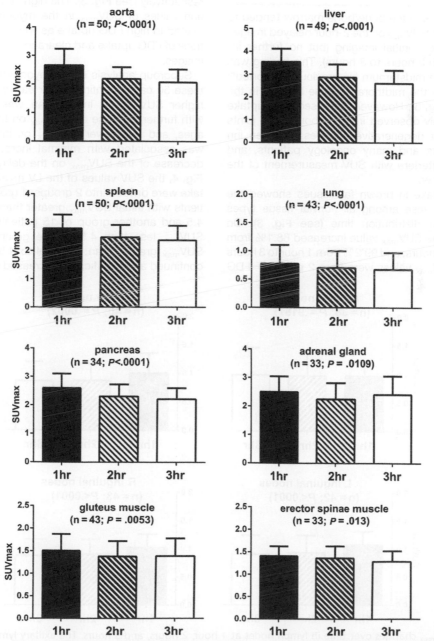

Fig. 1. SUV$_{max}$ changes over time in various tissues. The SUV$_{max}$ values for each tissue are graphed at 1 hour, 2 hours, and 3 hours. There is decrease in activity over time. Error bar, standard deviation; N, number of cases.

delay images (**Fig. 2**). The SUV_{max} was higher on the delay images in many cases. It is postulated that tracer injection resulted in more or less injection infiltration at the injection site, and that continued draining of the activity from the infiltration kept the FDG activity higher in the axillary nodes on the injection side compared with the lymph nodes elsewhere.

Tissues with Increased FDG Uptake on Delayed Images

FDG uptakes in the bone/bone marrow tended to have higher SUV_{max} on the 2-hour delayed images versus 1-hour initial imaging (but no further increase from 2 hours to 3 hours). This finding was noted in the midsternum (as previously reported[9]) and also in the midthoracic spine but not in the sacrum (**Fig. 3**). However, increased FDG uptake is commonly observed in many bones and joints because of degenerative changes, as seen inn our patients and many oncology patients, and this may interfere with SUV measurement of the bone marrow.

FDG uptake in brown fat tissues showed the largest increase among all normal tissue types with longer distribution time (see **Fig. 3**). On average, the SUV_{max} value increased 68.1% from 1 hour to 2 hours, and 99.2% from 1 hour to 3 hours (all 20 SUV_{max} values were from 2 patients). FDG

uptake in brown fat tended to be intense on the initial 1-hour images. Even so, multiple additional foci of brown fat activity were visualized on the delayed images, which were not included in this analysis (because of uncertainty in obtaining initial low SUV_{max} values).

In most cases, FDG uptake in the LV myocardium was intense, with progressively increased activity at sequential time points. The average values of myocardial SUV_{max} were 10.23, 12.54, and 14.05, at 1-hour, 2-hour, and 3-hour delays, respectively (see **Fig. 3**). The high standard deviation values of SUV_{max} in the myocardium were related to high FDG uptake as well as large variations of FDG uptake and clearance on the delayed images.

Subgroup analysis of the myocardial uptake in these 50 cases confirmed our earlier finding that higher SUV_{max} on initial scan was associated with further increase of SUV_{max} on the delay images, and that lower SUV_{max} on initial imaging was associated with minimal increase or even decrease of the SUV_{max} on the delay images. In **Fig. 4**, the SUV values of the LV myocardium uptake were divided into 2 groups: 1 group of 35 patients with initial SUV_{max} greater than or equal to 4.5 and another group of 15 patients with initial SUV_{max} less than 4.5. In the group with initial SUV_{max} greater than or equal to 4.5, there was continued and significantly increased FDG uptake

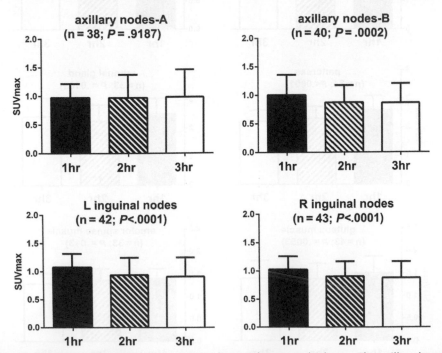

Fig. 2. SUV_{max} changes over time in lymph nodes at 1 hour, 2 hours, and 3 hours. The axillary lymph nodes are divided into A and B. A, injection side; B, contralateral side to the injection. The inguinal nodes are divided in to the left (L) and right (R). Error bar, standard deviation.

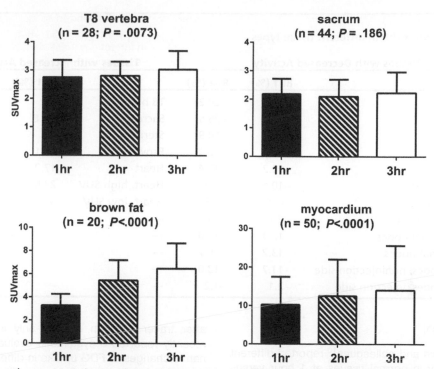

Fig. 3. SUV$_{max}$ changes over time in various tissues at 1 hour, 2 hours, and 3 hours. Error bar, standard deviation.

(RI, 52.3%) on the 3-hour delay images. In the group with initial SUV$_{max}$ less than 4.5, 10 out of 15 cases showed decreased FDG uptake on the 3-hour-delay images (RI, −1.8%).

Tissues with Nonsignificant Changes in FDG Uptake on Delayed Images

FDG uptake in the parotid gland, thyroid gland, and prostate gland was more variable with no significant change in SUV value on delayed imaging, as described previously[9] (data not presented here).

RI and Implication for Clinical Practice: An Example

Table 1 summarizes the clearance of FDG activity in different tissue types, as expressed by RI.

Continued background clearance of FDG activity in most normal tissues indicates that delayed FDG-PET imaging may help to improve image quality. The liver is an ideal organ for such a purpose because its background activity clearance is greatest. An example is shown in **Fig. 5.** A 63-year-old man with lung cancer had a few foci of increased FDG uptake on initial FDG-PET scan. On 2-hour-delay (images not shown) and 3-hour-delay images, all these lesions had higher activity with a few additional FDG-avid lesions not seen on the initial images. The lesion/background (LTB) ratio (SUV$_{max}$ of a lesion/mean SUV of the liver) was 2.7 on the delay images compared with 1.6 on the initial images. There was a 75% increase of LTB ratio, although the increase of SUV$_{max}$ was only 29% from 1-hour-delay to 3-hour-delay images.

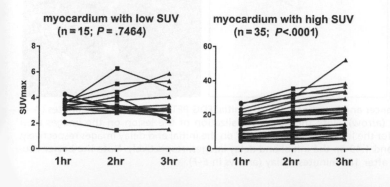

Fig. 4. SUV$_{max}$ changes over time in the LV myocardium in subjects with low FDG uptake (SUV$_{max}$<4.5) on the initial images versus moderate or high FDG uptake (SUV$_{max}$≥4.5) on the initial images. Error bar, standard deviation.

Table 1
Retention index (RI) in different tissue types

Tissues with Decreased Activity			Tissues with Increased Activity		
	RI-1 (%)	RI-2 (%)		RI-1 (%)	RI-2 (%)
Aorta	−16.6	−20.2	T8 bone	3.3	11.5
Liver	−19.0	−26.5	Sacrum	−3.8	1.4
Spleen	−11.1	−14.9	Sternum	6.5	9.3
Lung	−8.1	−12.3	Brown fat	68.1	99.2
Pancreas	−10.2	−13.4	Heart	17.2	26.9
Adrenal gland	−10.1	−2.9	Heart, high SUV	23.0	39.3
Gluteus muscle	−4.3	−3.3	Heart, low SUV	3.4	−1.8
Paraspinal muscle	−2.7	−7.6	—	—	—
Right inguinal nodes	−12.1	−14.0	—	—	—
Left inguinal nodes	−13.2	−16.7	—	—	—
Axillary nodes, noninjection side	−11.7	−13.0	—	—	—
Axillary nodes, injection side	−2.1	−1.2	—	—	—

DISCUSSION

In 2009, Chin and colleagues[10] reported different FDG activity in normal tissues at 1 hour versus 3 hours, using data obtained from one group for 1-hour-delay images and another group for 3-hour-delay images rather than serial determination of FDG uptake in 1 group of patients. Earlier, Kubota and colleagues[11] evaluated FDG activity in the lung, liver, and mediastinum at 1 and 2 hours after tracer injection on PET-only images. We recently reported a systematic evaluation of dynamic changes of FDG uptake in different normal tissue types with serial SUV quantification in one group of patients after single injection of FDG using a dedicated PET/CT system.[9] Additional data in this study reinforced our preliminary results that, although FDG uptake in some tissues decreases over time on delayed images, uptake

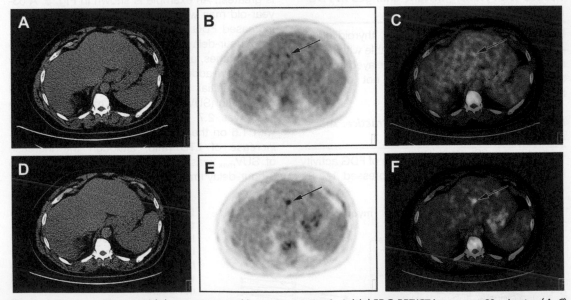

Fig. 5. A 63-year-old man with lung cancer and hepatic metastasis. Initial FDG-PET/CT images at 69 minutes (*A–C*) show a lesion with mild FDG uptake (*arrow*). Note the better visualization of the lesion on the images after 189 minutes' delay (*D–F*). The SUV$_{max}$ for the lesion was 3.24 and 4.17 on the initial and delay images respectively. The mean SUV for the liver was 1.99 and 1.49 on the initial and delay images, respectively. Note the better visualization of the lesion on the images after 189 minutes' delay (*arrows* in *E–F*).

may be stable or even increase over time in other tissues.

It is important to be familiar with the pattern of dynamic FDG uptake in PET imaging considering that FDG-PET image acquisition time can vary significantly in clinical practice. For the comparison of SUVs in 2 different studies, the imaging techniques ideally should be similar (including similar tracer distribution time), and SUV should be measured when an equilibrium phase has been reached if it is to be an accurate indicator of tissue FDG activity. However, this rarely happens because intracellular FDG accumulation changes constantly and varies for each tissue type.

For a similar reason, the current Society of Nuclear Medicine and Molecular Imaging procedure guideline of FDG-PET[1] lists optimal distribution time for FDG as an issue requiring further clarification.

The finding of continued background clearance in most tissues indicates that there is likely to be a higher signal/background ratio on delayed FDG-PET imaging, and that selective use of delayed imaging may increase sensitivity and specificity of an FDG-PET/CT study. In contrast, the differential clearance of background activity in different tissue types suggests that some tissues (with lower background level on delayed imaging) may be more suitable candidates than other tissues for delayed imaging. In the present study, background clearance in some tissues (including the blood pool, liver, and spleen) continued from 1 to 2 hours and from 2 to 3 hours, indicating that a longer distribution time may be helpful for these tissues. In contrast, background signal intensity in other tissues (lung, lymph nodes) did not decrease from 2 to 3 hours, indicating that delaying imaging beyond the 2-hour time point is not necessary in these tissues. Still other tissues (parotid, thyroid, and prostate) showed more stable FDG uptake over time, suggesting that delaying imaging is not likely to facilitate the detection of lesions in these tissues.

On dual-time-point imaging, the higher FDG activity is often used as an indication of positivity for malignancy. However, care should be taken to differentiate false-positive from true accumulation of FDG activity when using dual-time-point imaging. Our data showed that a higher SUV value was commonly visualized in the axillary nodes on the injection side, which should not be interpreted as a suspicious lymph node in a patient with breast cancer. Because the injection site in the forearm is often not included in the whole-body FDG-PET/CT images, the injection infiltration might be neglected. Another possible false-positive finding is small lymph node activity next to small and mild brown fat activity. The small and mild brown fat activity may not be attended on the initial images, but may be a cause of false-positive findings on delayed images. In addition, we noticed that there was significant overlap in SUV_{max} (heterogeneous FDG activity) for either the initial or delayed FDG-PET images, suggesting that it would be difficult to determine a cutoff value of SUV to define a normal versus abnormal value even on delayed imaging. Similar findings were observed in nonmalignant lesions[12] and in malignant lesions.[13] As a result, using a cutoff SUV_{max} value for the diagnosis of malignancy is not recommended.

Among all the tissues we analyzed, the liver had the greatest clearance of the FDG activity over time, likely because of the high expression level of glucose-6-phosphatase in hepatocytes.[14,15] Hence, delayed images of the liver improve the detection rate of hepatic lesions because of the background clearance over time.[7] In clinical practice, it is often to find relatively high and heterogeneous FDG uptake in the liver, which makes it difficult to evaluate small hepatocellular lesions of primary or metastatic disease.[16,17] Delayed FDG-PET imaging seems to be helpful for those, as reported in multiple studies,[11,18–22] not only because most malignant lesions tend to have 10% to 15% higher SUV value on delayed images but also because the continued background clearance in the liver tends to have 25% to 30% decrease in the background activity on delayed images. Combinations of these lead to approximately 40% to 50% increase in the LTB ratio on delayed images, which results in significantly increased imaging quality and diagnostic accuracy (as Dirisamer and colleagues[20] reported, up to 30% of all verified liver lesions could only be detected in the delayed FDG-PET images).

SUMMARY

The clearance of FDG activity in normal tissues (and thus the background level) varies significantly with extended distribution time. Although most tissues have lower SUV values on 2-hour/3-hour delayed images, others may have stable or higher FDG activity with longer distribution times. This finding has to be taken into consideration when interpreting an FDG-PET study that is performed with significantly short or long distribution time, and when comparing 2 studies with different distribution times. The continuously decreased SUV value from 1 to 3 hours in some tissues, especially in the liver, indicates that longer distribution time will decrease background activity and improve imaging quality, whereas the continuously increased

SUV values from 1 to 3 hours in the heart suggest that longer distribution time will improve detection of viable myocardium in a viability study.

ACKNOWLEDGMENTS

We thank Dr Martin Heyworth for valuable suggestions and recommendations during article preparation.

REFERENCES

1. Delbeke D, Coleman RE, Guiberteau MJ, et al. Procedure guideline for tumor imaging with 18F-FDG PET/CT 1.0. J Nucl Med 2006;47(5):885–95.

2. Juweid ME, Stroobants S, Hoekstra OS, et al. Use of positron emission tomography for response assessment of lymphoma: consensus of the Imaging Subcommittee of International Harmonization Project in Lymphoma. J Clin Oncol 2007;25(5):571–8.

3. Hustinx R, Smith RJ, Benard F, et al. Dual time point fluorine-18 fluorodeoxyglucose positron emission tomography: a potential method to differentiate malignancy from inflammation and normal tissue in the head and neck. Eur J Nucl Med 1999;26(10):1345–8.

4. Zhuang H, Pourdehnad M, Lambright ES, et al. Dual time point 18F-FDG PET imaging for differentiating malignant from inflammatory processes. J Nucl Med 2001;42(9):1412–7.

5. Matthies A, Hickeson M, Cuchiara A, et al. Dual time point 18F-FDG PET for the evaluation of pulmonary nodules. J Nucl Med 2002;43(7):871–5.

6. Alkhawaldeh K, Bural G, Kumar R, et al. Impact of dual-time-point (18)F-FDG PET imaging and partial volume correction in the assessment of solitary pulmonary nodules. Eur J Nucl Med Mol Imaging 2008; 35(2):246–52.

7. Cheng G, Torigian DA, Zhuang H, et al. When should we recommend use of dual time-point and delayed time-point imaging techniques in FDG PET? Eur J Nucl Med Mol Imaging 2013;40(5):779–87.

8. Higashi T, Saga T, Nakamoto Y, et al. Relationship between retention index in dual-phase (18)F-FDG PET, and hexokinase-II and glucose transporter-1 expression in pancreatic cancer. J Nucl Med 2002; 43(2):173–80.

9. Cheng G, Alavi A, Lim E, et al. Dynamic changes of FDG uptake and clearance in normal tissues. Mol Imaging Biol 2013;15(3):345–52.

10. Chin BB, Green ED, Turkington TG, et al. Increasing uptake time in FDG-PET: standardized uptake values in normal tissues at 1 versus 3 h. Mol Imaging Biol 2009;11(2):118–22.

11. Kubota K, Itoh M, Ozaki K, et al. Advantage of delayed whole-body FDG-PET imaging for tumour detection. Eur J Nucl Med 2001;28(6):696–703.

12. Cheng G, Alavi A, Del Bello CV, et al. Differential washout of FDG activity in two different inflammatory lesions: implications for delayed imaging. Clin Nucl Med 2013;38(7):576–9.

13. Suga K, Kawakami Y, Hiyama A, et al. Differential diagnosis between (18)F-FDG-avid metastatic lymph nodes in non-small cell lung cancer and benign nodes on dual-time point PET/CT scan. Ann Nucl Med 2009;23(6):523–31.

14. Caraco C, Aloj L, Chen LY, et al. Cellular release of [18F]2-fluoro-2-deoxyglucose as a function of the glucose-6-phosphatase enzyme system. J Biol Chem 2000;275(24):18489–94.

15. Keiding S. Bringing physiology into PET of the liver. J Nucl Med 2012;53(3):425–33.

16. Lin WY, Tsai SC, Hung GU. Value of delayed 18F-FDG-PET imaging in the detection of hepatocellular carcinoma. Nucl Med Commun 2005;26(4):315–21.

17. Wolfort RM, Papillion PW, Turnage RH, et al. Role of FDG-PET in the evaluation and staging of hepatocellular carcinoma with comparison of tumor size, AFP level, and histologic grade. Int Surg 2010; 95(1):67–75.

18. Nishiyama Y, Yamamoto Y, Fukunaga K, et al. Dual-time-point 18F-FDG PET for the evaluation of gallbladder carcinoma. J Nucl Med 2006;47(4):633–8.

19. Arena V, Skanjeti A, Casoni R, et al. Dual-phase FDG-PET: delayed acquisition improves hepatic detectability of pathological uptake. Radiol Med 2008;113(6):875–86.

20. Dirisamer A, Halpern BS, Schima W, et al. Dual-time-point FDG-PET/CT for the detection of hepatic metastases. Mol Imaging Biol 2008;10(6):335–40.

21. Lee JW, Kim SK, Lee SM, et al. Detection of hepatic metastases using dual-time-point FDG PET/CT scans in patients with colorectal cancer. Mol Imaging Biol 2011;13(3):565–72.

22. Fuster D, Lafuente S, Setoain X, et al. Dual-time point images of the liver with (18)F-FDG PET/CT in suspected recurrence from colorectal cancer. Rev Esp Med Nucl 2012;31(3):111–6.

Postradiation Changes in Tissues
Evaluation by Imaging Studies with Emphasis on Fluorodeoxyglucose-PET/ Computed Tomography and Correlation with Histopathologic Findings

Liran Domachevsky, MD[a,b], Heather A. Jacene, MD[a,b],
Christopher G. Sakellis, MD[a,b], Chun K. Kim, MD[b,*]

KEYWORDS

- Radiation • Postradiation change • Positron emission tomography/computed tomography
- Tolerance dose • Fluorodeoxyglucose • Tissue necrosis

KEY POINTS

- An optimal radiation treatment is one in which the tumor gets most of the radiation dose while sparing normal tissues.
- Radiation injury to tissue is classified as acute (hours to days or hours to months depending on the type of tissues/organs) or delayed (months to years) and is usually related to the time from the end of radiation to the appearance of morphologic changes or symptoms.
- The use of newer radiation techniques forces the imaging specialist to be familiar with radiation ports, radiation dose, and the time from the end or beginning of radiation therapy as these can become crucial to the correct interpretation of imaging studies.
- Fluorodeoxyglucose-PET/computed tomography might help to differentiae tumor recurrence from tissue necrosis.

INTRODUCTION

Radiation is a process in which energy is emitted in the form of particles or waves. Ionizing radiation refers to radiation with sufficient energy to strip an electron from an atom. The initial energy deposited by ionizing radiation can result in tissue damage. The effects of radiation on a tissue are dependent on the absorbed dose, type of radiation, and the radiosensitivity of the tissue. Soon after the discovery of radiography, investigators noticed tissue damage to the skin after prolonged exposure to the radiation. The potential use of this damage effect of radiation on cancer cells was realized, and the first attempted radiation treatment was in 1896 by Victor Despeignes on a patient with stomach cancer.[1]

Radiation therapy has since become a key component in the treatment of cancer. External X-ray beam radiation therapy is the most

a Department of Imaging, Dana-Farber Cancer Institute, 450 Brookline Avenue, Boston, MA 02215, USA;
b Division of Nuclear Medicine and Molecular Imaging, Department of Radiology, Brigham and Women's Hospital, Harvard Medical School, 75 Francis Street, Boston, MA 02115, USA
* Corresponding author.
E-mail address: ckkim@bwh.harvard.edu

PET Clin 9 (2014) 217–235
http://dx.doi.org/10.1016/j.cpet.2013.10.005
1556-8598/14/$ – see front matter © 2014 Elsevier Inc. All rights reserved.

commonly used; however, energy can be delivered in different ways, for example, proton beam radiation. In addition, the source of radiation can be located inside the body (eg, brachytherapy), adjacent to or within an area requiring treatment. Well-planned radiation therapy delivers a homogeneous radiation dose to a tumor, with minimal effect on normal tissues. Regardless, normal tissues within a radiation port may be affected.

The therapeutic ratio is defined as the tumor control probability/normal tissue complication probability (NTCP). Rubin and Cassarett[2] reported normal tissue tolerance doses (TDs) by using TD 5/5 and TD 50/5. TD 5/5 and 50/5 represent the 5% and 50% NTCP occurring within 5 years after radiotherapy, respectively, when an entire organ is irradiated. In cases in which a fractional volume of an organ is irradiated, TD50 is replaced by TD50v (partial volume-dependent parameter).[3] Normal tissue tolerance is affected by a spectrum of confounding parameters, which are related to the treatment, host, organ, and tumor type,[4] but a detailed discussion of this is beyond the scope of this article.

Radiation injury to tissue is classified as acute (hours to days or months, depending on the type of tissues/organs) or delayed (months to years) based on the time from the end (in most cases) of radiation therapy to the appearance of morphologic changes or symptoms. Postradiation changes seen in tissues are grouped into 3 categories: epithelial (parenchymal), stromal (mesenchymal), and vascular. Principal epithelial changes include atrophy, necrosis, ulceration, atypia, and dysplasia. Principal stromal changes include fibrosis, lack or paucity of cellular inflammatory exudate, atypical fibroblastic changes, and fibrinous exudate. Vascular changes differ with regard to the type and size of the involved vessel. Blood capillaries and sinusoids are the most radiosensitive. Changes in these vessels include damage to endothelial cells, ectasia, rupture, and thrombosis.[5]

In recent years, there have been tremendous efforts to minimize the damage incurred to adjacent normal tissues during radiotherapy, primarily by shifting from the use of conventional radiotherapy to more advanced techniques. Conventional radiotherapy uses a few simply shaped beams, usually directed in the anterior-posterior and posterior-anterior projections, which cover the area of the tumor. With this technique, irradiation of adjacent normal tissues is unavoidable. Newer techniques, such as three-dimensional conformal radiation therapy and stereotactic body radiation therapy, take advantage of the ability to image the tumor in 3 dimensions and to use multiple beam angles that conform to the shape of the tumor. Intensity-modulated radiotherapy permits variation in dose intensity within a single beam.[6]

Because postradiation changes in tissues have no pathognomonic features on imaging studies, it is crucial to be aware of patients' previous radiation therapy. The use of multiple beam angles with newer radiation techniques forces radiologists to be familiar with the radiation ports, the radiation dose, and the time from the end of radiation therapy, because these can be crucial for the correct interpretation of imaging studies. This article summarizes postradiation (primarily external beam) histologic findings as well as multimodality imaging findings, with an emphasis on [18F]fluoro-deoxyglucose (FDG)-PET/computed tomography (CT). Imaging findings related to internal radiotherapy are mentioned at the end.

EXTERNAL RADIOTHERAPY
Central Nervous System

Brain
Radiation has a crucial role in the treatment of primary and metastatic tumors in the brain as well as in the treatment of several benign conditions, such as arteriovenous malformation. Brain tissue might also be irradiated in a few head and neck cancers, such as nasopharyngeal cancers. Radiation-induced central nervous system injury is divided into acute (days to weeks after radiation), early-delayed (1–6 months after radiation) and late-delayed (>6 months after radiation) phases. Acute and early-delayed injuries are usually reversible, whereas late-delayed injury is permanent and progressive.[7]

Histopathologic features The end point of irreversible radiation injury to the brain is necrosis, mainly in the white matter, and demyelination.[7] The most significant predictive factors for the occurrence of tissue necrosis are the total dose and fractional dose.[8]

Imaging (non-PET) The primary modality for follow-up imaging of the brain is magnetic resonance (MR) imaging. Radiation necrosis may appear differently on MR imaging in different clinical settings.[8]

New brain abnormalities within the radiation port in a patient treated for head and neck malignancy are usually manifested as abnormal T2-weighted signal, mainly in the white matter. However, the gray matter may also be involved. Enhancing areas reflecting disruption of the blood-brain barrier can also be seen.[9] Given the very low prevalence of intracranial metastases from head and neck tumors, a new abnormal finding in brain tissue within the radiation port on MR imaging is more likely to represent radiation necrosis rather than a new primary brain lesion or metastasis.[10]

The second clinical setting involves radiation treatment of brain tumor. Radiation can be delivered in multiple fractions or as single precise high-dose radiation (stereotactic radiation). One of the morphologic changes in brain tumor after stereotactic radiation is a transient increase in size or increase in the extent of enhancement. These changes usually occur 3 to 12 months after treatment and tend to disappear 5 to 7 months after onset.[11] Differentiating persistent/recurrent tumor from radiation necrosis in this scenario is challenging. MR imaging parameters have been proposed in an attempt to differentiate between the 2 possibilities in this clinical setting (ie, lesion enlargement after radiosurgery). For example, the lesion quotient, defined as the ratio of the size of the nodule on T2 imaging to the size of the total enhancing area on T1 imaging, was found to be a reliable parameter for differentiating recurrent tumor from radiation necrosis.[12]

In the case of fractionated radiation therapy, there are several imaging findings on brain MR imaging supporting the diagnosis of radiation necrosis. These findings include new enhancing foci within and circumscribing a previously nonenhancing lesion as well as development of enhancing foci in the periventricular white matter and at sites distant from the primary tumor but within the radiation port.[13] Ruben and colleagues[14] found that the period between the completion of radiation therapy and the diagnosis of radiation necrosis was in the range of 2 to 32 months. Therefore, changes that appear 3 years after the end of radiation are more likely to represent tumor recurrence. Findings that are more suggestive of recurrent tumor include new enhancement next to the resection cavity and progressive increase in size with mass effect.[8]

FDG-PET Numerous studies assessed the value of FDG-PET or FDG-PET/CT for differentiating radiation necrosis from recurrent tumor. Several criteria have been adopted for this purpose.[15–19] However, the standardized uptake value (SUV) alone has not been widely used, which seems natural given the exceptionally wide variation in FDG avidity in brain tumors.[20]

Visual comparison of the lesion FDG uptake with surrounding brain tissue seems to be a simple and popular criterion.[15–17] However, the reported specificities using this criterion varied widely (ie, 62.5%, 81%, and 97%), although the sensitivities were within a narrow range (ie, 75%–82%). A plausible explanation for the wide range of specificities is the variation of the time intervals between radiation therapy and PET scanning. The range of the RT-PET interval was approximately 2 to 196 months in the study reporting the specificity of 97%,[17] and 1 to 39.3 months in the study reporting the 81% specificity.[15] Although the RT-PET interval was not specifically mentioned in the study reporting the 62.5% specificity,[16] the investigators state that all patients were symptomatic within 11 months after radiation. Given this statement and the context, it is conceivable that the RT-PET interval in this study might have been considerably shorter than those in the other 2 studies. If that is the case, the 3 reported specificities are certainly in line with the 3 RT-PETs interval. It is also uncertain whether or not other factors, such as variations in the radiotherapy protocol (eg, mode, dose) caused variation in the reported specificities.

Investigators using contralateral gray matter as the reference region found FDG-PET to be of limited value with a sensitivity of 73% and specificity of 56%.[18]

It has been shown that the tumor/nonirradiated brain ratio increases on delayed imaging in both primary[21] and metastatic brain lesions.[19] In patients with treated brain metastases and MR imaging findings suspicious for recurrence, Horky and colleagues[19] calculated the ratio of maximum SUV (SUVmax) between a lesion and contralateral frontal gray matter (at the level of the thalamus and the centrum semiovale), measured at approximately 1 and 4 hours (mean 3.8 hours, range 2–5.7 hours) after injection. These investigators reported that an increase of the lesion/gray matter ratio greater than 19% was 95% sensitive, 100% specific, and 96.4% accurate for distinguishing between tumor and radiation necrosis.

Wide variations exist in the criteria/parameters for the purpose of differentiating tumor recurrence from radiation necrosis in the brain. The results also vary among the studies using similar criteria. In general, the higher the FDG uptake, the more likely the diagnosis of tumor is, and vice versa (**Fig. 1**). However, there is significant overlap in FDG uptake between tumor and tissue necrosis, making the differential diagnosis challenging (**Fig. 2**). Because this is particularly more difficult in the early period after radiation, the recommendation is not to perform the study within 4 weeks after the end of radiation.[22]

There are some additional considerations. It has been reported that FDG uptake in the nonirradiated portion of the brain is also decreased (17% on average).[23] The impact of this result on some of the criteria using the nonirradiated brain as the reference region is unknown. Coregistration

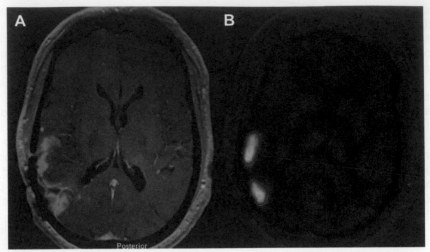

Fig. 1. Recurrent brain tumor in a 48-year-old man with recurrent anaplastic astrocytoma. (*A*) Axial MR image 4 years after radiation shows an enhancing mass in the right parietal and temporal lobes. (*B*) Fused FDG-PET/MR image shows intense FDG uptake, which corresponds to the enhancing areas on MR.

of the PET and MR imaging is reported to improve the sensitivity.[15]

Several other PET radiotracers, such as carbon-11-methionine,[24,25] [18F]fluoro-L-thymidine,[26] [18F]fluoroethyl-L-tyrosine[27] and [11C]choline,[16] have been examined, some with promising results. The usefulness of these tracers is not further discussed in this article.

Spinal cord

The human spinal cord consists of 31 segments. It tapers craniocaudally, except at the levels of cervical and lumbar enlargement at spinal levels C3-T2 and T9–12, respectively. The cervical enlargement gives rise to the spinal nerves that form the brachial plexus and the lumbar enlargement is the source of the lumbosacral plexus. There are 2

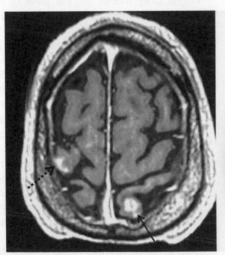
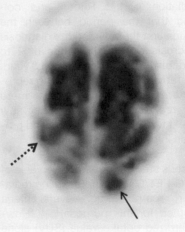

Fig. 2. Postradiation changes. A patient with a history of melanoma had FDG-PET and MR imaging examinations 10 months after radiation to the metastatic brain lesions. Postcontrast T1-weighted MR image showed enhancing foci in the left posterior parietal lobe (*solid arrow*) and in the right frontal lobe (*dotted arrow*). FDG uptake in these 2 areas is higher than immediately surrounding brain, which was also included in the radiation port, but lower than more anterior frontal gray matter. Both lesions would be interpreted as positive for tumor recurrence if either surrounding brain[15–17] or contralateral gray matter[18] is used as the reference standard. There was an approximately 15% to 20% increase in the lesion/contralateral frontal ratio (at the level of thalamus) between early and delayed imaging, which would be considered borderline negative according to Horky and colleagues'[19] criteria. This case shows a variation in the interpretation according to different criteria and the clinical dilemma often encountered. Follow-up studies showed no progression.

major distinct clinical syndromes involving the spinal cord after radiation. The first is Lhermitte syndrome, which is a self-limited, early-delayed reaction seen a few weeks to several months after radiation.[28] Lhermitte syndrome is characterized by a sensation similar to an electric shock passing down the spine in the craniocaudal direction, which is precipitated or worsened by neck flexion. The second syndrome is delayed myelopathy, which usually appears after a latent time of about 1 to 2 years. Patients usually present with sensory symptoms, which, in most cases, progress to permanent motor deficits.[29]

Histopathologic features Oligodendrocytes and vascular endothelial cells are probably the cells that are most affected by radiation. Pathologic findings of postradiation human myelopathy mainly comprise lesions involving the white matter parenchyma and the blood vessels (ie, extensive demyelination that progresses to white matter necrosis and intramedullary vascular damage progressing to hemorrhagic necrosis or major infarcts, respectively).[30]

Imaging (non-PET) Early MR imaging findings in the irradiated cord in patients with radiation myelopathy include low signal on T1-weighted images, high signal on T2-weighted images, and eccentric focal contrast enhancement. It has been reported that the site of eccentric focal contrast enhancement correlated with the clinical manifestations. Atrophy of the spinal cord is usually the only late finding.[31]

FDG-PET Do and colleagues[32] assessed FDG uptake in the spinal cord in patients with non–central nervous system malignancy. They found a pattern of decreasing FDG uptake in the spinal cord in the craniocaudal direction, with significant increases relative to other vertebral levels at the T11–12 level, and a mild increase, albeit insignificant, at the C4 level. This pattern of FDG uptake seems to correlate with the amount of neural tissue that is present within the spinal cord. Mean SUV in the spinal cord is reported to range from approximately 2.1 to 2.6 at the C1 level to 1.0 at the L5 level.[32,33]

Esik and colleagues[34] followed changes in FDG and [11C]methionine uptake in the spinal cord of a 49-year-old woman with early hypopharyngeal cancer treated with a spinal cord dose of 40 Gy. There was increased FDG uptake in the exposed cervical spinal cord 2 months after radiotherapy, which declined 7 months later and nearly reached the baseline level by 44 months after the completion of radiation therapy. No changes were seen in [11C]methionine uptake within the irradiated and the nonirradiated spinal cord.

Chest/Lungs

Radiation therapy to the lungs is used as definitive, adjuvant, and palliative treatment of various lung and nonlung cancers. Acute radiation-induced lung disease (RILD) appears within 6 months after the completion of radiation, with symptoms including cough, dyspnea, chest discomfort, and fever. The acute phase might resolve or progress into a late phase, which clinically presents as chronic dyspnea, dry cough, or even respiratory failure.[35] Factors that influence the potential degree of injury include patient age, radiation dose, the irradiated volume, irradiation technique, and previous or concomitant chemotherapy.[35,36] Based on a multivariate analysis, Graham and colleagues[37] found the percentage of total lung volume exceeding 20 Gy (V_{20}) to be the single independent predictor of pneumonitis of grade 2 or higher, with a strong correlation between V_{20} and the severity of pneumonitis.

Histopathologic features

Radiation-induced morphologic changes in the lung have been described as 3 consecutive phases: acute exudative, organizing/proliferative, and late. In the acute exudative phase, the capillary endothelial cells are affected, which leads to increased permeability and interstitial edema. This stage is followed by protein leakage and macrophage infiltration in the organizing/proliferative phase. In the late phase, there is increased collagen deposition.[35,38]

Imaging (non-PET)

The imaging modality of choice for evaluating radiation-induced pulmonary changes is CT. In the acute phase, there is perivascular haziness, followed by ground-glass opacities or consolidation in the radiation portal (**Fig. 3**). Occasionally, an ipsilateral pleural effusion (**Fig. 4**) associated with atelectasis may develop. The acute phase might resolve (**Fig. 5**) or progress into the chronic phase. In the chronic phase, traction bronchiectasis, linear scarring, volume loss, and consolidation are seen. Consolidation usually has a sharp border, which conforms to the radiation portal. In general, radiation fibrosis is seen as parenchymal consolidation with a straight lateral margin and air bronchograms. Occasionally, these findings are associated with ipsilateral displacement of the mediastinum and adjacent pleural thickening or effusion (**Fig. 6**). Radiation fibrosis usually develops within 6 to 24 months, after which it tends to remain stable.[35,39]

The differentiation between posttreatment changes and residual/recurrent disease can be difficult. Radiographic signs supporting the

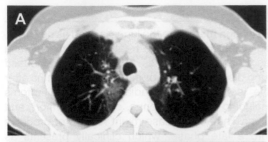

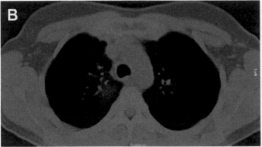

Fig. 3. Radiation pneumonitis in a 23-year-old woman with history of Hodgkin lymphoma after chemotherapy, autologous stem cell transplantation, and posttransplant consolidative radiation to the neck and mediastinum. (*A*) CT image of the lungs 9 months after completion of radiation shows paramediastinal ground-glass opacities that correspond to the radiation port. (*B*) Axial fused FDG-PET/CT image shows diffuse, low-level FDG-avid ground-glass opacities.

diagnosis of tumor recurrence include homogeneous opacities without air bronchograms, convex rather than straight borders, and filling in of bronchi within an area of radiation fibrosis.[40]

FDG-PET
Increased FDG uptake can be seen in radiation pneumonitis, and, therefore, it is generally

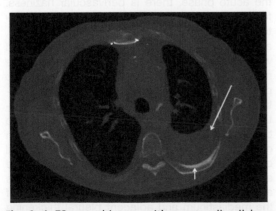

Fig. 4. A 72-year-old man with non–small cell lung cancer of the left posterior basal segment, after radiation to the left lower lobe to a dose of 60 Gy. Axial CT image obtained 5 months after completion of radiation shows pleural effusion (*long arrow*) and periosteal reaction (*short arrow*) in the anterior aspect of the left posterior rib.

recommended to wait at least 3 months after the completion of radiation to perform FDG-PET/CT.[41] After this time, increased FDG uptake is worrisome for residual/recurrent disease, especially if seen at the same location of the previous tumor. Low-level FDG uptake in the setting of RILD has a high negative-predictive value.[42] Changes occurring over a short period are less likely to represent malignancy and can be seen in infectious processes or in the context of steroid treatment discontinuation.[41]

Although FDG uptake is moderate to high, uptake with a sharply demarcated margin and geographic pattern corresponding to the radiation port typically represents postradiation changes (see also Fig. 18 in the article by Wachsmann and Gerbaudo elsewhere in this issue). However, using newer radiation therapy techniques, such as stereotactic radiotherapy, three-dimensional conformal radiation therapy, and intensity-modulated radiation therapy, multiple radiation beams are delivered to generate dose distributions that conform more tightly to target volumes compared with conventional radiation therapy. Thus, these techniques may result in focal radiation changes in a nongeographic pattern. Knowledge of the radiation modality as well as the dosimetry map is often helpful in these cases.

GASTROINTESTINAL SYSTEM
Esophagus

The esophageal wall consists of 4 layers: the mucosa, submucosa, muscularis propria, and adventitia. The superficial mucosal layer (epithelium) serves as a permeability barrier, whereas the deep layer (stratum basale) replenishes the epithelium. Acute esophagitis is a common side effect of radiotherapy for thoracic tumors.[43] The symptoms typically begin after the first 2 weeks of treatment and usually resolve within several weeks after completion of therapy.[44] Symptoms include dysphagia, odynophagia, and substernal burning pain. Late esophageal toxicity manifests as dysphagia associated with stricture or fistula, usually developing between 3 and 40 months after radiation.[45]

Histopathologic features
Most pathologic changes in the esophagus after radiation occur in the mucosa, because of the high rate of cell turnover, and include cytoplasmic vacuolization and absence of mitoses of the basal layer, followed by proliferation of the basal cells and regeneration of the epithelium. Late pathologic changes mainly involve the muscular layer.[46]

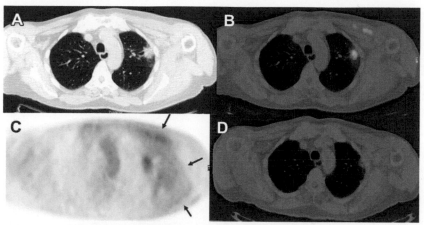

Fig. 5. Resolving radiation pneumonitis in a 75-year-old man with metastatic melanoma to a left axillary lymph node. (*A–C*) Axial CT, fused axial FDG-PET/CT, and axial PET images obtained 4 months after completion of radiation show mildly FDG-avid nodular consolidation in the left upper lobe. Note the diffuse mild FDG uptake in the adjacent soft tissue (*arrows*). (*D*) Fused PET/CT image obtained 12 months after completion of radiation shows an interval decrease in size and avidity of parenchymal changes.

Imaging (non-PET)

Double-contrast esophagography is used to evaluate postradiation esophageal complications. In the setting of acute esophagitis, granular appearance of the mucosa as well as small ulcers might be seen. In addition, esophageal narrowing within the radiation port is a common finding. Esophageal stricture is considered as a late esophageal complication and is usually seen radiographically with smooth and tapering borders.[47]

FDG-PET

On FDG-PET in healthy individuals, low-level FDG uptake can be seen in the distal esophagus and

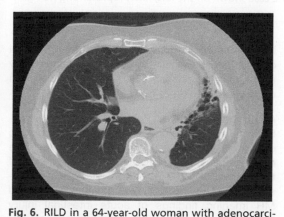

Fig. 6. RILD in a 64-year-old woman with adenocarcinoma of the left lower lobe of the lung. CT image obtained 8 months after completion of neoadjuvant radiation shows fibrotic changes, including traction bronchiectasis, volume loss, and leftward mediastinal shift. Note the sharp demarcation between normal lung tissue and areas of fibrosis.

may represent excreted FDG in swallowed secretions or smooth muscle activity.[48] Mild to moderately increased FDG uptake in the distal esophagus/gastroesophageal junction can also be seen in patients with gastroesophageal reflux and is secondary to inflammatory changes.[49]

Radiation esophagitis is usually seen as contiguous linear increased FDG uptake in the portion of the esophagus included in the radiation port.[50] The presumed radiation port is also associated with decreased FDG uptake in nearby vertebrae (**Fig. 7**). On the contrary, esophageal cancer frequently presents as focal intense FDG uptake (**Fig. 8**), particularly when it is associated with a mass on fused PET/CT images. However, detection of residual/recurrent esophageal cancer can be difficult in the presence of diffuse esophageal activity. In addition, SUV values can vary because of misregistration of the PET images and CT images. This variation is most pronounced at the distal esophagus and can result in variation in the calculated SUVmax of more than 50%.[51]

Stomach and Bowel

The stomach and small bowel are often incidentally irradiated when targeting tumors in the upper gastrointestinal tract, inferior lung, and retroperitoneum. The small bowel is also incidentally irradiated during radiation therapy to the pelvis. The terminal ileum is more commonly injured, because it is more fixed in location.[52] Toxicity is classified as acute when it occurs within 3 months of radiation therapy or as chronic when it occurs more than 3 months after

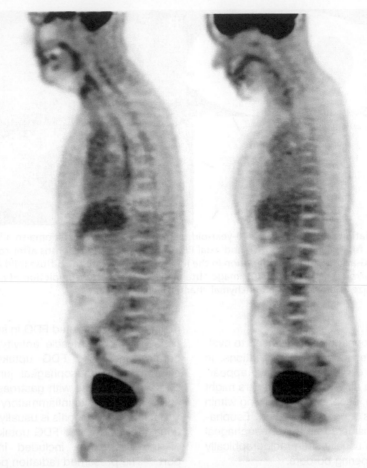

Fig. 7. (*Left*) Sagittal PET image obtained 6 months after completion of radiation to the lower neck and mediastinum shows diffusely increased FDG uptake in the esophagus and relatively decreased FDG uptake in the lower cervical and thoracic vertebrae, which were included in the radiation port. (*Right*) A 39-year-old woman with a history of nasopharyngeal carcinoma, status after radiation treatment 5 years previously. Sagittal PET image shows decreased FDG uptake in the cervical and upper thoracic vertebrae corresponding to the radiation portal. Esophageal uptake is not as significantly increased as in the case shown on the left, likely representing no significant ongoing inflammation.

therapy.[53] The incidence of toxicity depends on both therapy-related and patient-related factors. Factors such as previous surgery and preexisting vascular damage seem to be predictors of intestinal complications.[54] Therapy-related factors include radiation dose, the irradiated volume, and concomitant chemotherapy.[55] Symptoms of acute toxicity include nausea, abdominal pain, and diarrhea. Symptoms of chronic small bowel toxicity include persistent diarrhea, ulceration, fistula, perforation, bleeding, and malabsorption. Chronic stomach toxicity manifests as dyspepsia and ulceration.[55]

Histopathologic features
Early injury to the stomach presents as edema and degeneration of the mucosa, whereas late injury is caused by submucosal fibrosis.[52] Early intestinal injury is manifested as cell death in the intestinal crypt and villi. Chronic bowel injury is caused by submucosal vascular alteration and collagen deposition, leading to fibrosis.[56]

Imaging (non-PET)
Early injury to the stomach presents as prepyloric or pyloric ulcers seen on barium studies. Late injury manifests as narrowing and deformation of the antrum and the pylorus, which are best assessed by fluoroscopic examination.[52] CT and MR imaging findings of acute intestinal injury include nonspecific wall thickening, mucosal hyperemia, and adjacent fat stranding. Delayed complications include fibrotic strictures, tethering of bowel loops, and fistula.[56] These findings can be also be assessed by dynamic studies such as fluoroscopy.

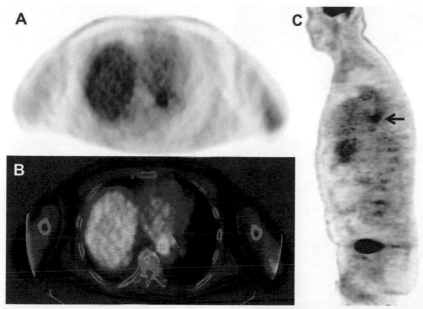

Fig. 8. An 82-year-old man with a long-standing history of gastroesophageal reflux disease and Barrett esophagus presented with newly diagnosed esophageal cancer. (*A, B*) Axial PET and fused FDG-PET/CT images show focal intense FDG uptake in the distal esophagus. (*C*) Sagittal PET image confirms the focal nature of the lesion (*arrow*).

FDG-PET

In healthy individuals, there is low to moderate uptake associated with the stomach, mostly in a diffuse pattern and typically involving the fundus. FDG uptake within the small and large bowel is highly variable. Patterns of physiologic bowel uptake range from diffuse low-level uptake to focal uptake.[49] Physiologic FDG uptake associated with the colon may be high, particularly in the cecum, ascending colon, and rectosigmoid regions.[57]

Radiation induces inflammatory changes and therefore increases FDG uptake. Metser and Even-Sapir[58] showed that when PET is performed 6 weeks after successful radiation therapy for cervical cancer, only mild FDG uptake is seen in pelvic bowel loops, likely indicating resolving radiation-induced inflammatory changes.

Rectum and Anus

The rectum and anus are fixed in position, which makes them vulnerable to radiation toxicity.[56] The rectum and anus might be irradiated in the setting of primary rectal cancer or when the rectum and anus are within the radiation port in the treatment of other pelvic cancers. Inflammation of the anus and rectum can occur in the acute or chronic setting. Acute radiation injury usually occurs approximately 2 weeks after starting therapy and increases in prevalence as treatment continues. The most common symptom is diarrhea. Other manifestations include abdominal pain, tenesmus, and, less commonly, rectal bleeding and nausea.[59] Chronic proctitis usually presents months to years after therapy (**Fig. 9**). Symptoms include rectal bleeding, mucous rectal discharge, urgency, rectal pain, and diarrhea.[60] Less commonly, patients may present with strictures or fistulas (**Figs. 10** and **11**).[52]

Histopathologic features

Changes in acute injury are usually limited to the mucosa, including the surface epithelium, glands, and lamina propria, manifesting as cryptitis, crypt abscess formation, and inflammation of the surface epithelium and lamina propria.[59] Chronic changes mainly involve the submucosa, with vascular abnormalities including focal distortion of small arteries as well as collagen proliferation in the submucosa.[46]

Radiation dose, fractionation, and radiation techniques affect the incidence of chronic proctitis. Several other factors that may influence the development of proctitis include younger age, previous abdominal surgery, and vasculopathy.[61]

Imaging (non-PET)

Acute radiation injury is usually manifested as mucosal irregularities seen on barium studies. MR imaging may show increased signal intensity of the rectal submucosa on T2-weighted images.

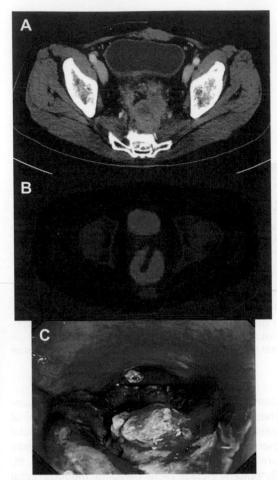

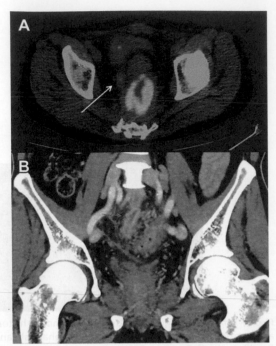

Fig. 10. The same patient as in **Fig. 9**. (*A*) Fused FDG-PET/CT image shows FDG-avid structure in the right pelvis adjacent to the bowel (*arrow*). (*B*) Coronal contrast-enhanced CT image shows an enhancing tubular tract. This structure extended from the sigmoid colon to the rectum consistent with a fistula (*arrow*).

Fig. 9. Radiation-induced proctitis in a 55-year-old man with history of rectal adenocarcinoma after neoadjuvant concurrent chemoradiation therapy. (*A*) Axial contrast-enhanced CT obtained 6 years after radiation shows severe thickening of the rectum associated with stranding of the perirectal fat. (*B*) Fused FDG-PET/CT image shows intense FDG uptake corresponding to thickened bowel wall on CT. (*C*) Endoscopy showed moderate inflammation characterized by friability.

Increased perirectal space and stranding of the perirectal fat are seen in the early and late phases. Wall thickening is usually seen as the injury progresses.[52]

FDG-PET

Kalff and colleagues[62] studied the effect of changes caused by external beam radiation on the restaging of patients with locally advanced rectal cancer by FDG-PET. Radiation changes were assessed visually and were compared with FDG uptake in tissues adjacent to the primary tumor on baseline evaluation, colonic uptake outside the radiation field, and nonrectal tissues within the

radiation port. Only 6% of the patients showed increased FDG uptake that was attributable to radiation. Higher FDG uptake was associated with inflammation on pathologic examination, whereas lower FDG uptake was associated with a small amount of residual disease. In the first 6 weeks after radiation, the time of imaging in relation to the end of radiation therapy did not affect the frequency of radiation changes.

GENITOURINARY SYSTEM
Kidneys

Radiation of the kidneys occurs if they are included within the radiation portal for the treatment of upper abdominal cancers or in total body irradiation in preparation for bone marrow transplantation (bone marrow transplantation nephropathy). Radiation nephropathy can also be seen after administrating hydrophilic radiolabeled peptides, which are filtered and retained within the kidneys.[63]

Radiation nephropathy is divided to acute (<3 months), subacute (3–18 months), and chronic (>18 months) phases. Acute radiation nephropathy occurs within 3 months of ending radiation and is generally subclinical.[64] In cases of bilateral renal radiation, symptoms and signs of nephropathy

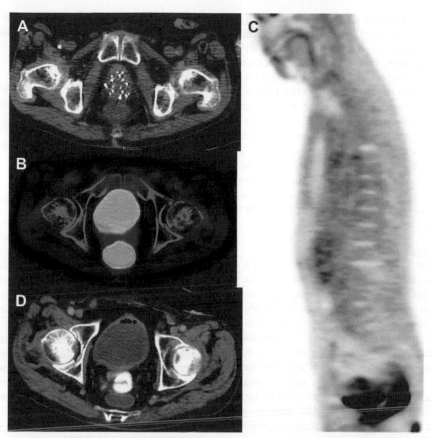

Fig. 11. Rectourethral fistula in a 78-year-old man with history of localized prostate cancer. (*A*) Axial CT image shows prostate brachytherapy seeds. (*B*) Fused FDG-PET/CT 8 years after placement of brachytherapy seeds shows intense FDG uptake in the rectum with SUV values similar to the urinary bladder. (*C*) Sagittal PET image shows the fistula between the urethra and the rectum. (*D*) Axial CT image shows air in the urinary bladder.

usually appear after 6 months. Symptoms include edema, dyspnea, and headache; signs include anemia, proteinuria, hypertension, and azotemia. Hypertension can be seen after unilateral renal radiation.[65]

Histopathologic features
It has been shown in animal models that both the glomeruli and the tubules are affected by irradiation, but that the glomerular changes appear earlier. Glomerular changes include abnormal capillaries and the presence of intercapillary eosinophilic material.[66]

Imaging (non-PET)
Imaging studies of radiation nephropathy are sparse because of the lack of clinical symptoms in the early stages. Wistow and colleagues[67] described increased technetium 99m methylene diphosphonate on bone scan, which began as focal uptake within the irradiated kidney 5 months after therapy and progressed to include all the irradiated kidney, correlating with the port edges,

6 months after radiation. A follow-up bone scan performed almost 10 months after radiation was normal. Ultrasonography and CT conducted 5 months after radiation were normal. Moore and colleagues[68] described a persistent nephrogram pattern on delayed-phase, contrast-enhanced CT images 3 months after the completion of radiation. The region that showed this pattern corresponded to the irradiated portions of the kidney. Later on, irradiated segments may show low attenuation, reflecting damaged tissue. Severe radiation injury to the entire kidney results in volume loss and atrophy.[52]

FDG-PET
To the best of our knowledge, there are no data in the literature regarding FDG uptake in irradiated kidney.

Bladder
Effects of radiation on the bladder are seen after treatments of bladder or pelvic malignancies and

may result from external or intracavitary radiation therapy. Doses and modes of radiation differ based on the type of malignancy and whether the bladder is specifically targeted (ie, bladder cancer) versus cases in which the bladder is located within the radiation port for the treatment of another tumor (eg, rectal cancer, cervical cancer). The clinical manifestations of radiation to the bladder are categorized into acute injury (during or within 3–6 months) and late injury. In the acute phase, symptoms usually include dysuria, urgency, and frequency. Late complications include decreased bladder capacity, cystitis, and bleeding. Less frequent complications include ulcer and fistula formation.[69]

Histopathologic features

Radiation was found to decrease the number of superficial urothelial cells and cause the loss of the normal protective glycosaminoglycan layer. This situation results in exposure of underlying tissues to hyperosmolar urine, which leads to inflammation and tissue damage.[70] Changes in endothelial cells can be seen as edema in the early stages or as hyperplasia, which appears later. Obliteration of blood vessels is a late manifestation. The bladder muscle is also affected by radiation, beginning with muscle cell edema and replacement of muscle cells by fibroblasts, leading to collagen deposition.[69]

Imaging (non-PET)

An inflamed bladder wall is seen on CT and MR imaging as thickening of the bladder wall accompanied by perivesicular fat stranding (**Fig. 12**). Increased T2-weighted signal of the bladder wall indicates edema. Mucosal hyperemia can also be seen. In the late phase, the urinary bladder appears small with thickened walls. Fistula formation, a less common complication, appears as a tubular structure connecting the bladder to adjacent structures. In the absence of bladder catheterization, gas within the bladder is an indirect sign of fistula.[71]

FDG-PET

Assessment of the urinary bladder wall with FDG-PET is challenging because of its proximity to physiologic FDG excreted within the urine. This intensely FDG-avid urine within the urinary bladder may falsely increase the SUV values as a result of partial volume effect.

SOLID ORGANS IN THE ABDOMEN
Liver

The liver is usually included in the radiation portal in the treatment of lower esophageal, gastrointestinal, pancreaticobiliary, or thoracolumbar spinal malignancies. Radiation-induced liver damage is a clinical syndrome characterized most commonly as hepatic dysfunction that is usually seen 2 weeks to 3 months after the completion of radiation, without evidence of progressive cancer within the liver. Patients present with hepatomegaly and ascites accompanied by marked increase of alkaline phosphatase levels and a modest increase in transaminases or bilirubin levels.[72]

Histopathologic features

Radiation injury to the liver probably begins with damage to the endothelial cells of central veins and sinusoids, which leads to sinusoidal congestion. In the more advanced stages, venoocclusive disease is seen, resulting in backflow congestion and liver necrosis.[72,73]

Imaging (non-PET)

In the acute phase, irradiated areas in the liver are hypodense compared with nonirradiated areas, unless the underlying liver is fatty, in which case the irradiated areas are hyperdense. On MR images, the irradiated area has increased signal on T2-weighted images. This phase corresponds to the sinusoidal congestion seen on histology, resulting in increased water content in the tissues. Because of alteration in blood flow, irradiated areas enhance to a lesser degree on the portal venous phase images (**Fig. 13**).[74] In most patients, these findings gradually resolve; however, in some cases, chronic changes appear, which include atrophy and fibrosis.[56]

FDG-PET

Although FDG uptake in the irradiated liver in a pig model has been reported to be decreased at 2 and 4 weeks after radiation,[75] changes in FDG uptake in the irradiated human liver seem

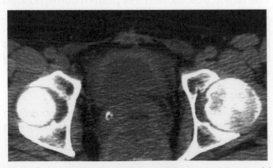

Fig. 12. Radiation-induced cystitis in a 55-year-old man with history of rectal cancer and radiation to the pelvis. Axial CT image shows thickening of the urinary bladder as well as adjacent fat stranding.

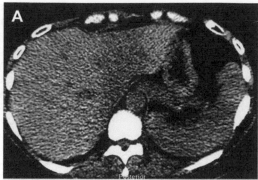

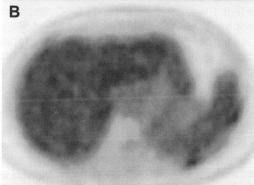

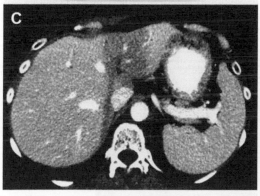

Fig. 13. Radiation-induced liver disease in a 53-year-old woman with metastatic breast cancer to the thoracic spine. (*A*) Axial CT image 1 month after completion of radiation shows straight border attenuation of liver parenchyma, which corresponds to the radiation port. (*B*) Axial FDG-PET shows no significant change or possibly a subtle increase in FDG uptake in the irradiated tissue. (*C*) Axial contrast-enhanced CT image better shows the demarcation lines between the irradiated and nonirradiated tissue.

to vary.[76] In a study including 26 patients whose left hepatic lobe was included within the radiation port,[76] FDG-PET performed 6 weeks after radiation showed no significant changes in the irradiated left lobe in 23 patients (in 2 of the 23 patients, unexplained increased uptake was seen in the nonirradiated right lobe), increased uptake in the irradiated left lobe in 2 patients,

and decreased uptake in both lobes in the remaining 1 patient. Increased FDG uptake in the irradiated left hepatic lobe has been shown in several other case reports.[77–79] It was suggested that such findings be interpreted with caution and correlated with other imaging, clinical, and laboratory findings to avoid confusion with hepatic metastases.

Spleen

Splenic irradiation can be used to alleviate symptoms caused by splenomegaly and hypersplenism in patients suffering from lymphoma and leukemia.[80] The spleen can also be included in the radiation port of malignancies located close to the spleen. Splenic irradiation has a direct local effect on neoplastic cells in the spleen but may also have systemic effects. Splenic tissue is very radiosensitive. Apoptosis of splenic cells can be seen with doses of as low as 0.05 to 0.5 Gy, whereas loss of splenic function has been reported to be associated with high overall doses higher than 20 Gy.[80] Doses in the range of 35 to 40 Gy may lead to splenic fibrosis.[74]

Imaging
To the best of our knowledge, there are no data in the literature regarding the appearance of irradiated spleen on imaging, other than atrophy seen on anatomic imaging studies.[81]

Pancreas

In the pancreas, the acinar cells are the most radiosensitive, followed by the duct cells and the islet cells. The relatively high sensitivity of acinar cells to radiation is manifested clinically as abnormal exocrine function.[82] It has been reported that radiation to the tail of the pancreas in children and young adults is associated with increased risk of developing diabetes in the future, which is likely related to the high concentration of islet cells in the tail of the pancreas.[83]

Histopathologic features
Early morphologic changes include reduced number of secretory granules in acinar cells. The ductal cells are affected to a lesser degree, whereas Langerhans islet cells appear normal. Late morphologic changes include fibrosis of the pancreatic parenchyma, decrease in the pancreas size, and loss of lobulation.[82]

Imaging
Imaging features resemble pancreatitis in the acute phase and may progress to atrophy.[84]

Adrenal Gland

The adrenal gland is not a radiosensitive organ, and adrenal failure is not reported as a complication of total body irradiation.[85]

BONE AND BONE MARROW

Mature bones are composed of extracellular organic and inorganic matrix, osteogenic cells, and blood cells. Blood cells are the most radiosensitive component.[86] In the immature bone, the physeal plate is most susceptible to radiation.[87] Radiation has a greater deleterious effect on osteoblasts than osteoclasts, resulting in overall high resorption/bone formation ratio, which results in decreased bone matrix density and puts patients at higher risk for pathologic fractures.[86]

Other clinical consequences of radiation include osteoradionecrosis and secondary bone tumors. In the growing bone, radiation causes growth disturbances and can result in short stature, scoliosis, kyphosis, and limb shortening.[82]

Histopathologic Features

Radiation injury to the bone is likely the result of damage to the cellular and vascular components.

A decrease in the number of vessels as well as obliterative endarteritis was seen after radiation. Although the osteoblasts are considered to be more radiosensitive than the osteoclasts, leading to bone resorption, several studies related bony changes to an increased number of osteoclasts or to impaired resorption and suggested that the remodeling process was mainly caused by osteoclast dysfunction.[87,88]

Imaging (non-PET)

On X-ray and CT, cortical osteopenia is often evident 1 year after radiation (Fig. 14). Bone formation on retained trabeculae occurs later and is seen as coarsened trabeculae. The radiographic appearance of mixed low-density and high-density areas is referred to as radiation osteitis.[87]

The earliest radiation-induced change on MR imaging is reported to be increased signal intensity on T2-weighted and short tau inversion recovery images that is believed to represent acute marrow edema, necrosis, and hemorrhage. This change is followed by an increase in signal intensity on T1-weighted images, which is compatible with fatty replacement of the bone marrow.[86]

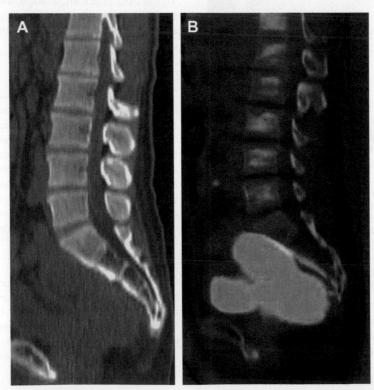

Fig. 14. Postradiation osteopenia in a 55-year-old man with a history of rectal cancer and pelvic irradiation. (A) Sagittal CT image obtained several years after radiation shows osteopenia of the sacrum. (B) Fused sagittal PET/CT image shows decreased FDG uptake in the sacrum.

FDG-PET

In a rodent model, Higashi and colleagues[89] found that FDG uptake in the irradiated bone marrow transiently increases, then decreases, and then returns to baseline. The initial increase of FDG uptake was associated with an influx of inflammatory cells into the irradiated area seen on marrow specimen examination. Most human FDG-PET studies performed several months after radiation typically show decreased FDG uptake in the bone marrow included in the radiation port (see **Figs. 7** and **14**). Rarely, there is persistent FDG uptake in the treated region years after radiation, which probably represents ongoing inflammation.[90]

Persistent high FDG uptake in irradiated bone can be seen in osteoradionecrosis.[91] The mandible is relatively more susceptible to radiation injury (**Fig. 15**). Osteoradionecrosis of the mandible is associated with doses higher than 60 Gy.[82]

INTERNAL RADIOTHERAPY

In this mode of therapy, the radiation source (usually radioisotopes) is located within or close to the tumor, resulting an increase in the therapeutic ratio. Therapeutic radioisotopes are administered in sealed or unsealed forms. Unsealed radioisotopes are given orally, intravenously, or may be placed directly into a body cavity. Examples include iodine 131 therapy for thyroid cancer and hyperthyroidism, [131I]metaiodobenzylguanidine for the treatment of pheochromocytoma and neuroblastoma, and radiolabeled anti-CD20 monoclonal antibodies such as [90Y]ibritumomab tiuxetan and [131I]tositumomab for the treatment of low-grade non-Hodgkin lymphoma. Most radioisotopes are β emitters, but several are α emitters, such as radium 223, which has recently been approved by the US Food and Drug Administration for the treatment of bone metastases from castrate-resistant prostate cancer. Sealed radiotherapy (also known as brachytherapy) uses radioisotopes that are enclosed in a protective capsule or wire and is used mainly in the treatment of prostate, cervical, and breast cancer.

Radioembolization

Yttrium 90 radioembolization is a catheter-based therapy, in which micrometer-sized radioactive particles are delivered transarterially into tumor microvasculture. This palliative therapy mode is used in unresectable primary and metastatic liver lesions and takes advantage of the predominance of arterial blood supply to hepatic tumors, thereby maximizing the therapeutic ratio. Yttrium 90 radioembolization treatment combines the benefits of internal radiation and the embolic effect of the microspheres. Yttrium 90 is a pure β emitter, with a mean tissue penetration of 2.5 mm before decaying to zirconium 90. Because the microspheres are trapped within the tumor microcirculation, tumors might receive doses as high as 150 Gy.[92]

Imaging (non-PET)

For radioembolization, posttreatment changes are mainly evaluated by CT and MR imaging. Findings include peritumoral edema and hemorrhage, ring enhancement (which is usually attributable to peripheral fibrous tissue and not to residual disease), and transient perivascular edema. Fibrotic changes can be seen in liver parenchyma and may cause capsular contraction and secondary portal hypertension. Although not common,

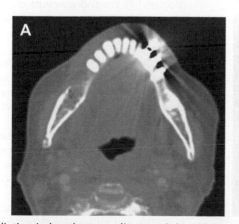
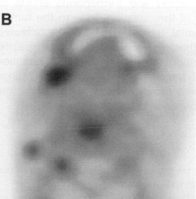

Fig. 15. Radiation-induced osteoradionecrosis in a 72-year-old woman with history of lymphoepithelial lesion of the nasopharynx after chemoradiation therapy. (*A*) Axial CT image shows a lytic lesion with cortical destruction in the right mandible. (*B*) Axial PET image shows increased FDG uptake, which correlates with the destructive lesion on CT.

adjacent structures such as the right pleura and liver capsule might be affected, manifesting as perihepatic fluid and pleural effusion.[93]

FDG-PET

FDG-PET was found to be helpful in assessing tumor response to treatment.[93] To the best of our knowledge, there are no data in the literature regarding FDG changes in the adjacent normal tissue.

Brachytherapy for Prostate Cancer

Twenty-five percent of patients with prostate cancer undergo radiation as a definitive treatment.[94] In brachytherapy, radioisotope particles, or seeds are implanted in the prostate gland. The most commonly used radioisotope is iodine 125.

Imaging (non-PET)

Posttreatment changes in the prostate gland are best characterized by MR imaging. Findings include a decrease in the size of the prostate gland, along with diffuse signal loss on T2-weighted images. There is also loss of zonal differentiation.[95]

FDG-PET

At present, FDG-PET and PET/CT are considered to have no significant role in the diagnosis of prostate cancer or in the evaluation of treatment response. To the best of our knowledge, there are no data in the literature regarding FDG changes in the prostate gland related to brachytherapy.

SUMMARY

Despite the significant advancement in radiation therapy techniques and tremendous efforts to deliver most of the radiation dose to the tumor, adjacent normal tissues may still be affected during radiotherapy. Familiarity with the specific type of radiation therapy, timing after radiation therapy, and the spectrum of imaging findings associated with radiation injury is crucial for the correct interpretation of imaging studies.

REFERENCES

1. Case JT. History of radiation therapy. Prog Radiat Ther 1958;1:13–41.
2. Rubin P, Cassarett G. A direction for clinical radiation pathology. In: Vaeth JM, Green JP, Schroeder AF, et al, editors. Frontiers of radiation therapy and oncology VI. Baltimore (MD): University Park Press; 1972. p. 1–16.
3. Emami B, Lyman J, Brown A, et al. Tolerance of normal tissue to therapeutic radiation. Int J Radiat Oncol Biol Phys 1991;21:109–22.
4. Milano MT, Constine LS, Okunieff P. Normal tissue tolerance dose metrics for radiation therapy of major organs. Semin Radiat Oncol 2007;17(2):131–40.
5. Fajardo LF. The pathology of ionizing radiation as defined by morphologic patterns. Acta Oncol 2005;44(1):13–22.
6. Nutting C, Dearnaley DP, Webb S. Intensity modulated radiation therapy: a clinical review. Br J Radiol 2000;73(869):459–69.
7. Tofilon PJ, Fike JR. The radioresponse of the central nervous system: a dynamic process. Radiat Res 2000;153(4):357–70.
8. Shah R, Vattoth S, Jacob R, et al. Radiation necrosis in the brain: imaging features and differentiation from tumor recurrence. Radiographics 2012;32(5):1343–59.
9. Chan YL, Leung SF, King AD, et al. Late radiation injury to the temporal lobes: morphologic evaluation at MR imaging. Radiology 1999;213(3):800–7.
10. de Bree R, Mehta DM, Snow GB, et al. Intracranial metastases in patients with squamous cell carcinoma of the head and neck. Otolaryngol Head Neck Surg 2001;124(2):217–21.
11. Friedman DP, Morales RE, Goldman HW. MR imaging findings after stereotactic radiosurgery using the gamma knife. AJR Am J Roentgenol 2001;176(6):1589–95.
12. Dequesada IM, Quisling RG, Yachnis A, et al. Can standard magnetic resonance imaging reliably distinguish recurrent tumor from radiation necrosis after radiosurgery for brain metastases? a radiographic-pathological study. Neurosurgery 2008;63(5):898–903 [discussion: 904].
13. Kumar AJ, Leeds NE, Fuller GN, et al. Malignant gliomas: MR imaging spectrum of radiation therapy– and chemotherapy-induced necrosis of the brain after treatment. Radiology 2000;217(2):377–84.
14. Ruben JD, Dally M, Bailey M, et al. Cerebral radiation necrosis: incidence, outcomes, and risk factors with emphasis on radiation parameters and chemotherapy. Int J Radiat Oncol Biol Phys 2006;65(2):499–508.
15. Chao ST, Suh JH, Raja S, et al. The sensitivity and specificity of FDG-PET in distinguishing recurrent brain tumor from radionecrosis in patients treated with stereotactic radiosurgery. Int J Cancer 2001;96(3):191–7.
16. Tan H, Chen L, Guan Y, et al. Comparison of MRI, F-18 FDG, and 11C-choline PET/CT for their potentials in differentiating brain tumor recurrence from brain tumor necrosis following radiotherapy. Clin Nucl Med 2011;36(11):978–81.

17. Wang SX, Boethius J, Ericson K. FDG-PET on irradiated brain tumor: ten years' summary. Acta Radiol 2006;47(1):85–90.

18. Ricci PE, Karis JP, Heiserman JE, et al. Differentiating recurrent tumor from radiation necrosis: time for re-evaluation of positron emission tomography? AJNR Am J Neuroradiol 1998;19(3):407–13.

19. Horky LL, Hsiao EM, Weiss SE, et al. Dual phase FDG-PET imaging of brain metastases provides superior assessment of recurrence versus post-treatment necrosis. J Neurooncol 2011;103(1): 137–46.

20. Kim CK, Alavi JB, Alavi A, et al. New grading system of cerebral gliomas using positron emission tomography with F-18 fluorodeoxyglucose. J Neurooncol 1991;10:85–91.

21. Spence AM, Muzi M, Mankoff DA, et al. 18F-FDG-PET of gliomas at delayed intervals: improved distinction between tumor and normal gray matter. J Nucl Med 2004;45:1653–9.

22. Kapoor V, Fukui MB, McCook BM. Role of 18F FDG PET/CT in the treatment of head and neck cancers: posttherapy evaluation and pitfalls. AJR Am J Roentgenol 2005;184(2):589–97.

23. Bruehlmeier M, Roelcke U, Amsler B, et al. Effect of radiotherapy on brain glucose metabolism in patients operated on for low grade astrocytoma. J Neurol Neurosurg Psychiatry 1999;66(5):648–53.

24. Tsuyuguchi N, Sunada I, Iwai Y, et al. Methionine positron emission tomography of recurrent metastatic brain tumor and radiation necrosis after stereotactic radiosurgery: is a differential diagnosis possible? J Neurosurg 2003;98:1056–64.

25. Ogawa T, Kanno I, Shishido F, et al. Clinical value of PET with 18F-fluorodeoxyglucose and L-methyl-11C-methionine for diagnosis of recurrent brain tumor and radiation injury. Acta Radiol 1991;32(3): 197–202.

26. Chen W, Cloughesy T, Kamdar N, et al. Imaging proliferation in brain tumors with 18F-FLT PET: comparison with 18F-FDG. J Nucl Med 2005; 46(6):945–52.

27. Galldiks N, Stoffels G, Filss CP, et al. Role of O-(2-(18)F-fluoroethyl)-L-tyrosine PET for differentiation of local recurrent brain metastasis from radiation necrosis. J Nucl Med 2012;53(9):1367–74.

28. Sheline GE, Wara WM, Smith V. Therapeutic irradiation and brain injury. Int J Radiat Oncol Biol Phys 1980;6(9):1215–28.

29. Dropcho EJ. Neurotoxicity of radiation therapy. Neurol Clin 2010;28(1):217–34.

30. Schultheiss TE, Stephens LC, Maor MH. Analysis of the histopathology of radiation myelopathy. Int J Radiat Oncol Biol Phys 1988;14(1):27–32.

31. Wang PY, Shen WC, Jan JS. Serial MRI changes in radiation myelopathy. Neuroradiology 1995;37(5): 374–7.

32. Do BH, Mari C, Tseng JR, et al. Pattern of 18F-FDG uptake in the spinal cord in patients with non-central nervous system malignancy. Spine (Phila Pa 1976) 2011;36(21):E1395–401.

33. Nakamoto Y, Tatsumi M, Hammoud D, et al. Normal FDG distribution patterns in the head and neck: PET/CT evaluation. Radiology 2005;234(3):879–85.

34. Esik O, Emri M, Szakáll S Jr, et al. PET identifies transitional metabolic change in the spinal cord following a subthreshold dose of irradiation. Pathol Oncol Res 2004;10(1):42–6.

35. Larici AR, del Ciello A, Maggi F, et al. Lung abnormalities at multimodality imaging after radiation therapy for non-small cell lung cancer. Radiographics 2011;31(3):771–89.

36. Claude L, Pérol D, Ginestet C, et al. A prospective study on radiation pneumonitis following conformal radiation therapy in non-small-cell lung cancer: clinical and dosimetric factors analysis. Radiother Oncol 2004;71(2):175–81.

37. Graham MV, Purdy JA, Emami B, et al. Clinical dose-volume histogram analysis for pneumonitis after 3D treatment for non small cell lung cancer. Int J Radiat Oncol Biol Phys 1999;45(2):323–9.

38. Gross NJ. The pathogenesis of radiation-induced lung damage. Lung 1981;159(3):115–25.

39. Park KJ, Chung JY, Chun MS, et al. Radiation-induced lung disease and the impact of radiation methods on imaging features. Radiographics 2000;20(1):83–98.

40. Bourgouin P, Cousineau G, Lemire P, et al. Differentiation of radiation-induced fibrosis from recurrent pulmonary neoplasm by CT. Can Assoc Radiol J 1987;38(1):23–6.

41. Choi YW, Munden RF, Erasmus JJ, et al. Effects of radiation therapy on the lung: radiologic appearances and differential diagnosis. Radiographics 2004;24(4):985–97.

42. Patz EF Jr, Lowe VJ, Hoffman JM, et al. Persistent or recurrent bronchogenic carcinoma: detection with PET and 2-[F-18]-2-deoxy-D-glucose. Radiology 1994;191(2):379–82.

43. Werner-Wasik M, Paulus R, Curran WJ Jr, et al. Acute esophagitis and late lung toxicity in concurrent chemoradiotherapy in patients with locally advanced non-small cell lung cancer: analysis of the Radiation Therapy Oncology Group (RTOG) database. Clin Lung Cancer 2011;12(4):245–51.

44. Antonadou D, Coliarakis N, Synodinou M, et al. Randomized phase III trial of radiation treatment +/-amifostine in patients with advanced-stage lung cancer. Int J Radiat Oncol Biol Phys 2001;51(4): 915–22.

45. Ahn SJ, Kahn D, Zhou S, et al. Dosimetric and clinical predictors for radiation-induced esophageal injury. Int J Radiat Oncol Biol Phys 2005;61(2): 335–47.

46. Coia LR, Myerson RJ, Tepper JE. Late effects of radiation therapy on the gastrointestinal tract. Int J Radiat Oncol Biol Phys 1995;31(5):1213–36.

47. Collazzo LA, Levine MS, Rubesin SE, et al. Acute radiation esophagitis: radiographic findings. AJR Am J Roentgenol 1997;169(4):1067–70.

48. Skehan SJ, Brown AL, Thompson M, et al. Imaging features of primary and recurrent esophageal cancer at FDG PET. Radiographics 2000;20(3): 713–23.

49. Kostakoglu L, Hardoff R, Mirtcheva R, et al. PET-CT fusion imaging in differentiating physiologic from pathologic FDG uptake. Radiographics 2004; 24(5):1411–31.

50. Bhargava P, Reich P, Alavi A, et al. Radiation-induced esophagitis on FDG PET imaging. Clin Nucl Med 2003;28(10):849–50.

51. Pan T, Mawlawi O, Nehmeh SA, et al. Attenuation correction of PET images with respiration-averaged CT images in PET/CT. J Nucl Med 2005;46(9):1481–7.

52. Capps GW, Fulcher AS, Szucs RA, et al. Imaging features of radiation-induced changes in the abdomen. Radiographics 1997;17(6):1455–73.

53. Andreyev J. Gastrointestinal complications of pelvic radiotherapy: are they of any importance? Gut 2005;54(8):1051–4.

54. Potish RA. Importance of predisposing factors in the development of enteric damage. Am J Clin Oncol 1982;5(2):189–94.

55. Kavanagh BD, Pan CC, Dawson LA, et al. Radiation dose-volume effects in the stomach and small bowel. Int J Radiat Oncol Biol Phys 2010; 76(Suppl 3):S101–7.

56. Maturen KE, Feng MU, Wasnik AP, et al. Imaging effects of radiation therapy in the abdomen and pelvis: evaluating "innocent bystander" tissues. Radiographics 2013;33(2):599–619.

57. Pandit-Taskar N, Schöder H, Gonen M, et al. Clinical significance of unexplained abnormal focal FDG uptake in the abdomen during whole-body PET. AJR Am J Roentgenol 2004;183(4):1143–7.

58. Metser U, Even-Sapir E. Increased (18)F-fluorodeoxyglucose uptake in benign, nonphysiologic lesions found on whole-body positron emission tomography/computed tomography (PET/CT): accumulated data from four years of experience with PET/CT. Semin Nucl Med 2007;37(3):206–22.

59. Hovdenak N, Fajardo LF, Hauer-Jensen M. Acute radiation proctitis: a sequential clinicopathologic study during pelvic radiotherapy. Int J Radiat Oncol Biol Phys 2000;48(4):1111–7.

60. Garg AK, Mai WY, McGary JE, et al. Radiation proctopathy in the treatment of prostate cancer. Int J Radiat Oncol Biol Phys 2006;66(5):1294–305.

61. Tagkalidis PP, Tjandra JJ. Chronic radiation proctitis. ANZ J Surg 2001;71(4):230–7.

62. Kalff V, Ware R, Heriot A, et al. Radiation changes do not interfere with postchemoradiation restaging of patients with rectal cancer by FDG PET/CT before curative surgical therapy. Int J Radiat Oncol Biol Phys 2009;74(1):60–6.

63. Vegt E, de Jong M, Wetzels JF, et al. Renal toxicity of radiolabeled peptides and antibody fragments: mechanisms, impact on radionuclide therapy, and strategies for prevention. J Nucl Med 2010;51(7): 1049–58.

64. Dawson LA, Kavanagh BD, Paulino AC, et al. Radiation-associated kidney injury. Int J Radiat Oncol Biol Phys 2010;76(Suppl 3):S108–15.

65. Cassady JR. Clinical radiation nephropathy. Int J Radiat Oncol Biol Phys 1995;31(5):1249–56.

66. Stephens LC, Robbins ME, Johnston DA, et al. Radiation nephropathy in the rhesus monkey: morphometric analysis of glomerular and tubular alterations. Int J Radiat Oncol Biol Phys 1995; 31(4):865–73.

67. Wistow BW, McAfee JG, Sagerman RH, et al. Renal uptake of Tc-99m methylene diphosphonate after radiation therapy. J Nucl Med 1979;20(1):32–4.

68. Moore L, Curry NS, Jenrette JM 3rd. Computed tomography of acute radiation nephritis. Urol Radiol 1986;8(2):89–91.

69. Marks LB, Carroll PR, Dugan TC, et al. The response of the urinary bladder, urethra, and ureter to radiation and chemotherapy. Int J Radiat Oncol Biol Phys 1995;31(5):1257–80.

70. Jaal J, Dörr W. Radiation-induced damage to mouse urothelial barrier. Radiother Oncol 2006; 80(2):250–6.

71. Wong-You-Cheong JJ, Woodward PJ, Manning MA, et al. From the archives of the AFIP: inflammatory and nonneoplastic bladder masses: radiologic-pathologic correlation. Radiographics 2006;26(6):1847–68.

72. Pan CC, Kavanagh BD, Dawson LA, et al. Radiation-associated liver injury. Int J Radiat Oncol Biol Phys 2010;76(Suppl 3):S94–100.

73. Sempoux C, Horsmans Y, Geubel A, et al. Severe radiation-induced liver disease following localized radiation therapy for biliopancreatic carcinoma: activation of hepatic stellate cells as an early event. Hepatology 1997;26(1):128–34.

74. Kwek JW, Iyer RB, Dunnington J, et al. Spectrum of imaging findings in the abdomen after radiotherapy. AJR Am J Roentgenol 2006;187(5): 1204–11.

75. Antoch G, Kaiser GM, Mueller AB, et al. Intraoperative radiation therapy in liver tissue in a pig model: monitoring with dual-modality CT-PET. Radiology 2004;230:753–60.

76. Iyer RB, Balachandran A, Bruzzi JF, et al. PET/CT and hepatic radiation injury in esophageal cancer patients. Cancer Imaging 2007;7:189–94.

77. Nakahara T, Takagi Y, Takemasa K, et al. Dose-related fluorodeoxyglucose uptake in acute radiation-induced hepatitis. Eur J Gastroenterol Hepatol 2008;20(10):1040–4.

78. Wong JJ, Anthony MP, Lan Khong P. Hepatic radiation injury in distal esophageal carcinoma: a case report. Clin Nucl Med 2012;37(7):709–11.

79. DeLappe EM, Truong MT, Bruzzi JF, et al. Hepatic radiation injury mimicking a metastasis on positron-emission tomography/computed tomography in a patient with esophageal carcinoma. J Thorac Oncol 2009;4(11):1442–4.

80. Weinmann M, Becker G, Einsele H, et al. Clinical indications and biological mechanisms of splenic irradiation in chronic leukaemias and myeloproliferative disorders. Radiother Oncol 2001;58(3): 235–46.

81. Charnsangavej C, Cinqualbre A, Wallace S. Radiation changes in the liver, spleen, and pancreas: imaging findings. Semin Roentgenol 1994;29:53–63.

82. Shrieve DC, Loeffler JS. Human radiation injury. Philadelphia, PA: Lippincott Williams & Wilkins; 2011. p. 441–3.

83. de Vathaire F, El-Fayech C, Ben Ayed FF, et al. Radiation dose to the pancreas and risk of diabetes mellitus in childhood cancer survivors: a retrospective cohort study. Lancet Oncol 2012; 13(10):1002–10.

84. Iyer R, Jhingran A. Radiation injury: imaging findings in the chest, abdomen and pelvis after therapeutic radiation. Cancer Imaging 2006;6:S131–9.

85. Kauppila M, Koskinen P, Irjala K, et al. Long-term effects of allogeneic bone marrow transplantation (BMT) on pituitary, gonad, thyroid and adrenal function in adults. Bone Marrow Transplant 1998; 22(4):331–7.

86. Williams HJ, Davies AM. The effect of X-rays on bone: a pictorial review. Eur Radiol 2006;16(3): 619–33.

87. Bluemke DA, Fishman EK, Scott WW Jr. Skeletal complications of radiation therapy. Radiographics 1994;14(1):111–21.

88. Dhakal S, Chen J, McCance S, et al. Bone density changes after radiation for extremity sarcomas: exploring the etiology of pathologic fractures. Int J Radiat Oncol Biol Phys 2011;80(4):1158–63.

89. Higashi T, Fisher SJ, Brown RS, et al. Evaluation of the early effect of local irradiation on normal rodent bone marrow metabolism using FDG: preclinical PET studies. J Nucl Med 2000;41(12):2026–35.

90. Silverman ED, Carson WK. Persistent F-18 deoxyglucose and Tc-99m methylene diphosphonate uptake in a lower extremity radiation port. Clin Nucl Med 2008;33(4):299–300.

91. Morag Y, Morag-Hezroni M, Jamadar DA, et al. Bisphosphonate-related osteonecrosis of the jaw: a pictorial review. Radiographics 2009;29(7):1971–84.

92. Lewandowski RJ, Salem R. Yttrium-90 radioembolization of hepatocellular carcinoma and metastatic disease to the liver. Semin Intervent Radiol 2006; 23(1):64–72.

93. Atassi B, Bangash AK, Bahrani A, et al. Multimodality imaging following 90Y radioembolization: a comprehensive review and pictorial essay. Radiographics 2008;28(1):81–99.

94. Cooperberg MR, Broering JM, Carroll PR. Time trends and local variation in primary treatment of localized prostate cancer. J Clin Oncol 2010; 28(7):1117–23.

95. Vargas HA, Wassberg C, Akin O, et al. MR imaging of treated prostate cancer. Radiology 2012;262(1): 26–42.

Fluorodeoxyglucose Positron Emission Tomography/ Magnetic Resonance Imaging
Current Status, Future Aspects

Rajan Rakheja, MD[a],*, Hersh Chandarana, MD[b],
Fabio Ponzo, MD[b], Alexandra L. Seltzer, MD[b],
Luis S. Beltran, MD[b], Christian Geppert, PhD[c],
Kent P. Friedman, MD[b]

KEYWORDS

- Positron emission tomography • Magnetic resonance • Sodium fluoride
- Apparent diffusion coefficient • Lung cancer • Bone metastases • Dementia

KEY POINTS

- In 2011 a new whole-body PET/magnetic resonance (MR) hybrid scanner (mMR Biograph, Siemens, Germany) that allows simultaneous MR and PET imaging was approved by the US Food and Drug Administration for human use.
- We hypothesize that PET/MR will be particularly powerful for situations in which PET/computed tomography is limited because of suboptimal anatomic resolution, including head and neck cancer, thyroid cancer, lung cancer with chest wall invasion, hepatocellular cancer, liver lesion characterization, gynecologic malignancies, and anorectal cancer.
- PET attenuation correction in simultaneous PET/MR is performed via a 20-second breath-hold MR attenuation correction map using a T1-weighted Dixon-based segmentation model.
- One of the strengths of PET/MR will lie in the evaluation of patients with dementia, because both modalities provide complementary information and allow for diagnosis of mixed dementias and superimposed diseases.
- Although it is believed that MR can be more sensitive for smaller bone metastases, PET can be more specific for differentiating benign from malignant lesions, and thus, there is potential for PET/MR to be superior for the assessment of osseous metastases than either modality individually.

INTRODUCTION

In 2011 a whole-body PET/magnetic resonance (MR) hybrid system based on simultaneous MR and PET acquisition (mMR Biograph, Siemens, Germany) was approved by the US Food and Drug Administration for human use. Although current clinical experience is preliminary, hybrid PET/MR is a promising technology for whole-body evaluation of oncology patients as well as focused examinations for various indications. Hybrid PET and MR imaging allows for simultaneous acquisition of PET and MR image data for optimal temporally matched anatomic and physiologic data and use of MR for attenuation correction.

We hypothesize that PET/MR will be particularly powerful in applications for which PET/computed

---

[a] Department of Nuclear Medicine/Radiology, Royal University Hospital, Saskatoon, Saskatchewan, Canada;
[b] Department of Radiology, New York University School of Medicine, 550 First Avenue, New York, NY, USA;
[c] MR R&D Collaborations, Siemens Healthcare, New York, NY, USA
* Corresponding author. Division of Nuclear Medicine, Department of Radiology, Tisch Hospital, 560 First Avenue, 2nd Floor, New York, NY 10016.
E-mail address: rajan.rakheja@gmail.com

PET Clin 9 (2014) 237–252
http://dx.doi.org/10.1016/j.cpet.2013.10.007
1556-8598/14/$ – see front matter © 2014 Elsevier Inc. All rights reserved.

tomography (CT) is limited because of suboptimal anatomic resolution; some examples include head and neck cancers, thyroid cancer, lung cancer with chest wall invasion, liver lesion characterization, gynecologic malignancies, and anorectal cancer. Quantitative multiparametric imaging comparing PET with diffusion, perfusion, and other parameters may improve diagnosis and management of disease.

PET/MR CAMERA BASICS

PET/MR design concepts have evolved over time; the first was a separate PET and MR gantry linked by a single sliding bed, the second was a PET/CT scanner combined with a separate MR equipped with a cross-modality compatible stretcher, and most recently a fully integrated system with a PET detector inside an MR imaging bore. This third design is the foundation for the Biograph mMR, which is used at our institution.

The major difference in the PET camera in the integrated PET/MR system compared with standard PET/CT cameras is that standard photomultiplier tubes are replaced by avalanche photodiodes for MR compatibility. Each block detector consists of 64 crystal elements and each crystal measures $4 \times 4 \times 20$ mm. In each ring there are 56 block detectors, and 64 detector element rings are arranged on the z-axis. The PET has a transaxial field of view of 59.4 cm and an inner detector ring diameter of 65.6 cm. The MR is equipped with a 3.0 T magnet featuring a state-of-the-art gradient and radiofrequency system (**Fig. 1**).

SUMMARY

- Three basic designs of PET/MR exist, including (1) separate systems based on PET/CT and MR with a cross-compatible stretcher, (2) separate PET and MR gantries connected by a single sliding bed, and (3) a

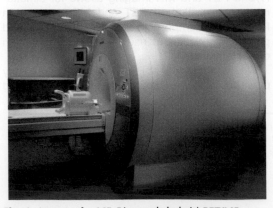

Fig. 1. Image of mMR Biograph hybrid PET/MR.

fully integrated system based on a PET detector inside an MR imaging bore.
- The principal difference in the PET camera in the integrated PET/MR system compared with PET/CT is that standard photomultiplier tubes are replaced by avalanche photodiodes for MR compatibility.

PET/MR IMAGING TECHNIQUE

Although early in our research program, we have imaged more than 150 PET/MR patients with various primary malignancies. Whole-body PET/MR is feasible and can be accomplished in approximately 45 to 70 minutes. PET and MR data are acquired simultaneously. Standard bed positions include head/neck, thorax, abdomen, and pelvis, with other areas depending on the malignancy and stage of disease. More focused examinations have also been performed, with the most common being brain PET/MR for evaluation of dementia and epilepsy.

For each bed, an approximately 20-second breath-hold MR-based attenuation correction map is acquired using a T1-weighted Dixon-based segmentation model (background, lungs, fat, soft tissue). Immediately afterward, the diagnostic MR sequences are performed, depending on the application. One of our common MR protocols for the abdomen includes coronal T2 turbo spin echo (TSE), fat-saturated T2-weighted, T1-weighted gradient echo imaging, and transverse diffusion-weighted imaging (DWI). These images are acquired simultaneously with PET data during free breathing. Imaging time is approximately 6 to 10 minutes for each bed position; however, further specific MR sequences require more time than just a basic set of sequences.

SUMMARY

- Attenuation correction is performed via a 20-second breath-hold MR attenuation correction map using a T1-weighted Dixon-based segmentation model
- Whole-body PET/MR is feasible and can be accomplished in approximately 45 to 70 minutes
- More focused studies are performed for specific indications, such as brain PET/MR for evaluation of dementia and epilepsy

PET/MR REPORTING

PET/MR is a complex, rapidly evolving hybrid modality, which in our opinion should be read by physicians with extensive experience in PET/CT and also MR imaging. This level of expertise may be achieved via joint reading sessions between experienced PET/CT readers (nuclear medicine physicians or radiologists) and subspecialists in MR imaging (body imagers for oncology cases, neuroradiologists for brain cases). A single reader may be possible if they have extensive experience in both PET/CT and MR imaging for the organ system being studied (brain, cardiac, or body MR based on current applications). It is a task for the national imaging societies to develop appropriate training criteria for performance and interpretation of PET/MR as the clinical applications evolve. Combined specialized training for nuclear medicine physicians and radiologists in certain areas of MR (brain imaging, body imaging) and nuclear medicine/PET may be required to optimally use this technology to benefit patients.

SUMMARY

PET/MR should be interpreted by physicians with experience in both PET/CT and MR, either as joint reading sessions or with single readers with advanced skills in PET and MR imaging.

CLINICAL APPLICATIONS
PET/MR in Lung Cancer

Lung cancer is the second most common malignancy in the United States and is responsible for the most cancer-related deaths in developed countries.[1] Staging with contrast-enhanced computed tomography (CT) is an important initial step in the management of patients who have lung cancer. CT usually includes the adrenals, given the high incidence of adrenal metastases. Patients with locally advanced disease undergo a brain MR imaging for assessment of intracranial metastases and, in some cases, bone scintigraphy (BS) (with either sodium fluoride [NaF]-PET or technetium Tc [99]m methylene diphosphonate [MDP]) to evaluate for skeletal metastases.[2] Although thoracic CT is mandatory for initial anatomic staging, it has several limitations: low

accuracy for differentiating obstructive atelectasis from tumor,[3] limited detection of metastases in normal-sized lymph nodes, and a failure to distinguish reactive hyperplasia from neoplasia.[4] PET/CT can overcome these difficulties and has now become a standard in the United States for staging of patients who have lung cancer.

Although PET/CT is an excellent staging modality, PET/MR may provide additional information about local staging as well as distant metastasis. Chest wall invasion is crucial presurgical information for the thoracic surgeon; unexpected chest wall disease can increase duration of surgery and add significantly to the complexity of the procedure.[5] MR may be able to more precisely identify chest wall invasion. In a study in which CT was unable to show definite chest wall involvement, Akata and colleagues[6] showed that respiratory-gated MR identified all patients with chest wall invasion. Other studies have also shown that MR could be more sensitive than CT for chest wall assessment; T2-weighted MR images were more reliable than CT for confirming tumor invasion of the soft tissue of the chest wall.[7,8] Early research has suggested PET/MR will be beneficial for lung cancer staging (**Fig. 2**).[9]

Similarly, PET/CT is a powerful lung cancer staging tool for assessment of mediastinal nodes.[10,11] Given the superior soft tissue resolution of mediastinal structures on MR, integrated PET/MR may offer superior diagnostic accuracy of mediastinal nodal involvement. The combination MR and PET/CT interpretation has been described by Kim and colleagues,[12] who reported that sensitivity for detecting nodal metastasis increased by combined interpretation to 69% from 46% for PET/CT alone. Moreover, there was no noted decrease in specificity.

Only one-third of patients with non-small cell lung cancer (NSCLC) who undergo curative surgical resection survive 5 years.[13] It is critical to exclude patients with distant metastases from invasive thoracotomies, thus minimizing patient anguish and unnecessary postsurgical

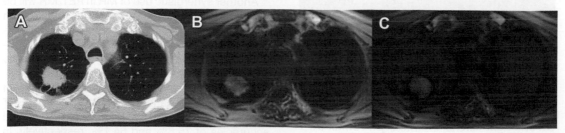

Fig. 2. A 63-year-old man with an intensely FDG-avid right upper lobe mass with pleural tethering on CT (*A*) and on PET/MR (*B*) T1 radial VIBE, (*C*) fused PET/T1 radial volumetric interpolated breath-hold examination.

comorbidities. Extrathoracic metastatic disease is usually a contraindication to surgery. Adrenal metastases are common, and 60% of patients with NSCLC develop adrenal metastases.[14] Although PET/CT is useful for evaluation of equivocal adrenal lesions, there are a few pitfalls, which may be overcome by PET/MR. Hemorrhage and necrosis are known to cause false-negative results in PET, and lipid-poor adenomas can mimic metastases on PET/CT. MR imaging can improve diagnosis of adenoma by detecting intravoxel fat. Furthermore, with use of gadolinium contrast and subtraction imaging, MR can improve evaluation of hemorrhagic lesions. In a study by Honigschnabl and colleagues,[15] the sensitivity, specificity, and accuracy of MR imaging for the differentiation of benign and malignant adrenal masses was 89%, 99%, and 93.9%, respectively (**Fig. 3**).

SUMMARY

- Early research has suggested that PET/MR will be beneficial for lung cancer staging
- Integrated PET/MR may offer superior diagnostic accuracy for local chest wall invasion and mediastinal nodal involvement
- MR can likely improve characterization of adrenal lesions in patients with lung cancer

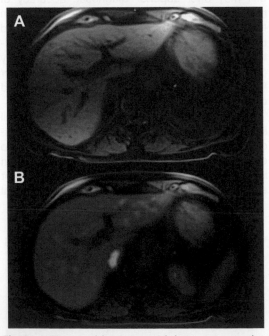

Fig. 3. A 65-year-old woman with lung cancer and an FDG-avid right adrenal metastases on PET/MR (*A*) T1 radial VIDE and (*B*) fused PET/radial volumetric interpolated breath-hold examination.

PET/MR AND DWI FOR ABDOMINAL/PELVIC MALIGNANCIES AND METASTASES

It is likely that PET/MR will be useful for abdominal/pelvic lesion characterization, given the superior contrast resolution of MR imaging. This benefit will be particularly relevant for local staging of primary malignancies in which PET/CT is limited, for example gynecologic malignancies, such as cervical and endometrial cancer.[16] Furthermore, with PET/MR, metabolic data from PET can be synergistically combined with DWI and dynamic contrast-enhanced MR imaging.

DWI is based on measuring the restriction to diffusion of water molecules within tissues. Neoplastic cells have more macromolecular proteins and larger nuclear/cytoplasmic ratios, resulting in restricted diffusion of water molecules and decreased apparent diffusion coefficient (ADC) values.[17] PET activity and DWI may serve as synergistic composite biomarkers; for example, 1 study[18] found that a combination of PET and DWI might increase diagnostic performance for differentiation between benign and malignant cervical lymph nodes (**Fig. 4**).

Our early PET/MR experience has shown us some examples of the superior soft tissue lesion characterization of neoplastic lesions in the abdomen/pelvis. For example, MR is an excellent modality for the detection of pancreatic lesions, an area in which noncontrast CT has some limitations. MR has been shown to be more sensitive than CT for the detection of pancreatic cancer.[19] Some research has also shown MR to be superior to PET for detection of malignant pancreatic lesions; Belião and colleagues[20] confirmed that the diagnostic accuracy of MR for the differential diagnosis of pancreatic lesions was 74% to 89%, compared with 67% for PET/CT. Conventional MR imaging combined with DWI provides beneficial information for the characterization of solid and cystic pancreatic neoplasms. Given the superior image contrast in DWI sequences, DWI may confirm small neoplastic implants better than PET/CT, and the strength of DWI is shown in **Fig. 5**.

Another synergistic use of MR in PET/MR will be for the evaluation of the liver; MR has been shown to be more sensitive for detection of liver metastases. Sahani and colleagues[21] studied the performance of enhanced liver MR and whole-body [18F]fluorodeoxyglucose (FDG)-PET for the detection of liver metastases from adenocarcinoma of the colon and pancreas. MR and FDG-PET showed sensitivities of 81.4% and 67.0% and accuracies of 75.5% and 64.1%, respectively. In addition, all subcentimetric lesions were identified

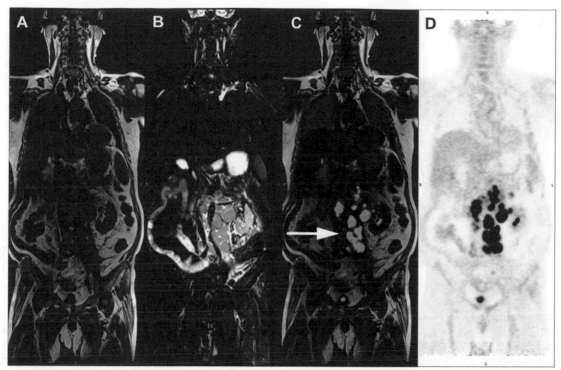

Fig. 4. FDG-PET/MR with coronal T1 (*A*), short tau inversion recovery (*B*), fused PET/T1 (*C*) and PET (*D*) images showing intensely FDG-avid enlarged lymphomatous abdominal nodes (*arrows*).

on MR, whereas less than half were detected on PET (**Fig. 6**).

SUMMARY

- PET/MR will allow for superior soft tissue lesion characterization of neoplastic lesions in the abdomen/pelvis

- MR and DWI will permit further characterization of nonspecific hypermetabolic findings in the liver, adrenals, and pancreas

HEAD AND NECK CANCERS

We envision that PET/MR will be useful for head and neck cancer, in terms of delineating local

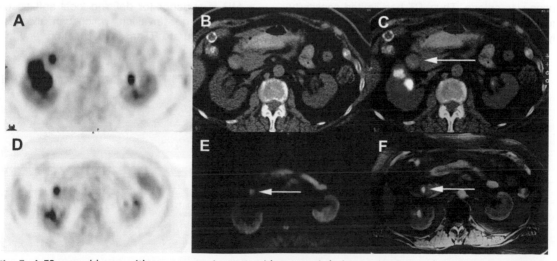

Fig. 5. A 52-year-old man with sarcoma and a FDG-avid metastatic lesion projecting to the pancreaticoduodenal groove on PET (*A* and *D*), CT (*B*), fused PET/CT (*C*), poorly seen on CT and clearly demarcated on DWI image with restricted diffusion (*E, arrow*) and on fused PET/T1 radial volumetric interpolated breath-hold examination (*F*). This case shows the superior soft tissue contrast of PET/MR for pancreatic lesions.

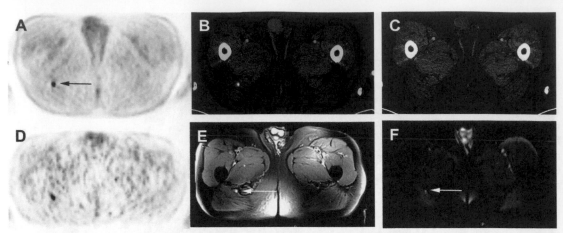

Fig. 6. A 54-year-old man with melanoma and an FDG-avid intramuscular deposit in the right gluteus maximus (*arrows*) on PET, fused PET/CT, and CT (*A–C*) without CT correlate. PET/MR (*D*) shows the focus as a T2 bright (1E–T2 blade) intramuscular metastases with restricted diffusion (1F, DWI), showing the superior soft tissue contrast of PET/MR.

tumor extent and for nodal involvement. Loeffelbein and colleagues[22] described the superior anatomic soft tissue resolution of closely associated anatomic structures with MR as an advantage over CT. These investigators showed that post-contrast T1-weighted images with fat saturation can more accurately delineate tumor margins. Earlier research has shown that fused images of PET/CT and MR allow for better target delineation in planning radiotherapy (RT) and in assessing disease recurrence.[23]

Although CT does provide precise anatomic information with high resolution, it suffers from a lower sensitivity/specificity for the presence or extent of nodal involvement, because it mainly uses size criteria. Thus, CT has limited sensitivity for metastases to nodal disease in normal-sized lymph nodes.[24] PET/MR will likely play an important role in excluding nonspecific enlarged neck nodes.[25] In addition, MR is superior for defining local osseous invasion, as opposed to superimposed osseous infection, which are ongoing limitations of CT.[25] The superior sensitivity of PET for detection of local disease and malignant neck nodes combined with the excellent anatomic resolution of MR can create the ideal hybrid imaging modality for head and neck malignancies (**Fig. 7**).

SUMMARY

- PET/MR will be extremely useful for head and neck malignancies, in terms of delineating local tumor extent and for nodal involvement
- MR is superior for defining local soft tissue and osseous invasion, which can allow for more accurate RT target delineation

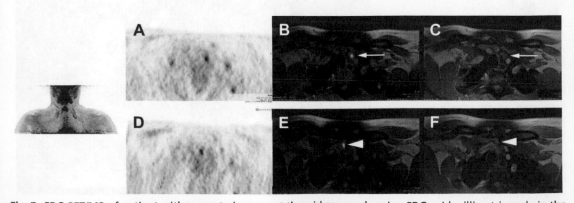

Fig. 7. FDG-PET/MR of patient with suspected recurrent thyroid cancer showing FDG-avid millimetric node in the left neck level IV (*arrow*) on PET (*A*), fused PET/radial volumetric interpolated breath-hold examination (VIBE) (*B*) and radial VIBE (*C*). A second tiny FDG-avid node anterior to left brachiocephalic vein (*D*, PET; *E*, fused PET/radial VIBE; *F*, radial VIBE), showing the superior soft tissue resolution of PET/MR.

PET/MR FOR EVALUATION OF OSSEOUS METASTASES: FDG- AND NAF-PET/MR

MR

MR imaging provides excellent contrast between a metastatic lesion and normal, healthy fatty bone marrow. On T1-weighted MR images, a metastasis in the bone marrow has a long T1 relaxation time and low signal intensity, which is in contrast to the high signal of the surrounding fatty tissue, resulting in high lesion conspicuity (see **Fig. 1**). On T2-weighted MR imaging, the relaxation times of metastatic lesions are variable. Tumor areas with a high density of cells show an intermediate signal intensity in T2-weighted imaging, whereas tumor areas with low cell density, such as areas of tumor necrosis after treatment, show high T2 relaxation times, with a significant increase in signal. In the setting of a metastatic lesion that stimulates surrounding osteoblasts and bone regeneration, there is a decrease in the T2 relaxation time, leading to a low signal intensity of the lesion. When T2-weighted sequences are supplemented with fat-suppression MR techniques such as an inversion pulse (short tau inversion recovery [STIR]) or frequency selective, there is higher contrast between the lesion and normal healthy fatty bone marrow compared with conventional T2-weighted imaging, thereby increasing lesion detection.[26]

Whole-body rapid MR has been technically feasible in a reasonable examination time since the advent of 1.5-T and 3-T MR systems.[27] Moreover, MR has been shown to have a high sensitivity for detection of osseous metastases; Buhmann-Kirchhoff and colleagues[28] showed that MR was significantly more sensitive for the detection of vertebral metastases (98.5%) compared with multidetector CT (MDCT), which had sensitivity of 66.2%. Specificity was not significantly different for both methods, with MDCT at 99.3% and MR at 98.9%. A meta-analysis[29] comparing the diagnostic performance of MR with different nuclear medicine methods in the detection of bone metastasis in more than 15,000 patients has provided the broadest data; both FDG-PET/CT and MR showed extremely high sensitivities and specificities and were significantly more accurate for bone metastasis detection than bone scans and CT.

Not only are PET and MR extremely sensitive modalities for bone metastases detection, they can be complementary. In a lesion-by-lesion analysis performed between whole-body MR and FDG-PET/CT for the detection of skeletal metastases, whole-body MR showed a superior sensitivity compared with PET/CT, because it could detect smaller lesions. However, specificity was higher for PET/CT (80% vs 76% for whole-body MR), because the metabolic information showed better discrimination between malignant and benign lesions.[30] Therefore, we believe that PET/MR will provide overall superior diagnostic accuracy for osseous metastases detection.

FDG-PET/CT

Recently, the effectiveness of BS in confirming or excluding malignant bone disease has been questioned, because skeletal metastases in the bone marrow can be detected with MR before scintigraphic detection.[31–33] In contrast to MR and CT, FDG-PET/CT provides both anatomic and metabolic information by localizing and quantifying increased glucose uptake in tumor cells. FDG-PET/CT for oncologic staging is highly sensitive for detection of bone metastases. For staging of lung cancer skeletal metastases, FDG-PET has a sensitivity of 98% and specificity of 95%. FDG-PET performs better than BS in the detection of early marrow metastases and lytic lesions **(Fig. 8)**.[34]

NAF-PET/MR IN PROSTATE CANCER

Ninety percent of patients with metastatic prostate cancer have bone metastases, and this is the only site of known disease in up to 70% of cases. Bone metastases may result in blood dyscrasias, cord compression, fracture, pain, neurologic compromise, and death. Therefore, early detection and accurate assessment of bone metastasis is of high clinical importance in management of patients with high-risk prostate cancer. The predominantly hematogenous spread of bone metastases explains their primary localization in the axial skeleton. However, up to 40% of bone metastases occur in the appendicular skeleton, and therefore, there is a need for whole-body anatomic imaging.[35]

^{99m}Tc-MDP BS is the standard method for initial bone metastases screening.[36] However, BS has only limited spatial resolution, and at the early stage of disease, bone metastases may remain undetected given their low metabolic activity or pure lytic characteristic. Furthermore, uptake seen on BS is nonspecific, and false-positive findings are frequently caused by healing fractures or degenerative disease. When scintigraphic findings have no radiographic correlate or when they are in anatomically complex regions, further evaluation with CT is usually required.

The role of FDG-PET in patients with prostate cancer is still under investigation, but lower sensitivities compared with BS have been reported,

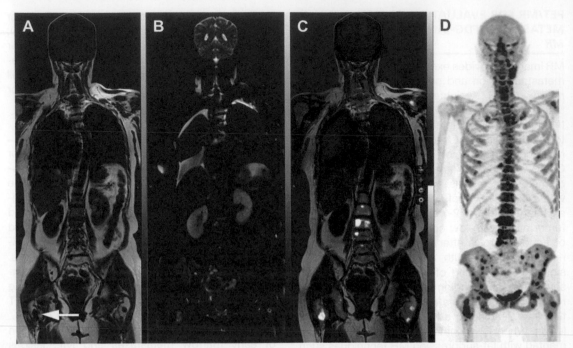

Fig. 8. A 66-year-old man with prostate cancer and several osseous metastases. [¹⁸F]NaF-PET/MR shows the superior bone marrow resolution of PET/MR; [¹⁸F]NaF-avid right proximal femoral metastases (*arrow*) correlating to hypointense signal on T1 TSE (*A*), increased signal on STIR (*B*), and intensely avid lesion on fused NaF/T1 TSE (*C*) and on NaF (*D*).

likely related to the low glucose metabolism of well-differentiated prostate cancer.[36,37] There is more promise for [¹⁸F]NaF bone scanning coupled with CT images, in view of its highly sensitive, three-dimensional anatomic and functional imaging of the skeleton.

[¹⁸F]Fluoride is a bone-seeking positron-emitting agent, has a 2-fold higher bone uptake than ⁹⁹mTc-MDP, a faster blood clearance, and a better target/background ratio.[38–40] [¹⁸F]Fluoride reflects the metabolic response of bone tissue to the presence of metastases, an indirect measurement of tumor activity. Given its high diagnostic accuracy, [¹⁸F]fluoride PET/CT has been recommended as a second bone-seeking agent to enhance diagnostic sensitivity for skeletal metastases in patients who have prostate cancer.[41] [¹⁸F]fluoride PET/CT has been reported to have a significantly higher sensitivity compared with planar and single-photon emission CT (SPECT) BS for the detection of skeletal metastases in prostate cancer.[36]

A recent study by Mosavi and colleagues[42] compared whole-body DWI and [¹⁸F]NaF-PET/CT in 49 high-risk patients who have prostate cancer. These investigators showed that DWI had a higher specificity but lower sensitivity than NaF-PET/CT and concluded that NaF-PET/CT is a sensitive study for detection of prostate osseous

metastases. We speculate that the combination of the superior MR bone marrow resolution with the excellent sensitivity of NaF-PET may provide the potential for a highly accurate hybrid imaging modality.

With the recent introduction of molecularly targeted therapies, including those that specifically target bone microenvironment,[43] some of these treatments can cause tumor flare, which appears as a worsening bone scan despite significant tumor cell death. This phenomenon limits the clinical usefulness of scintigraphy, thus creating a need for more accurate imaging modalities to assess treatment response to new molecular therapies for metastatic prostate cancer. Combined PET and MR data may provide complementary information in evaluating biological activity and treatment response of tumor, particularly using DWI.

DWI is of use in quantitatively assessing the response of bone metastases to systemic therapy, as has been shown for osseous prostate cancer metastases treated with antiandrogens.[44] DWI enables calculation of the tissue ADC, a quantitative measure of tissue diffusivity conventionally using 2 or more diffusion sensitizing gradients, referred to as b values. This technique allows objective analysis in oncology applications, such as in evaluating the tumor ADC before and after chemotherapy to identify treatment response. The calculated ADC value is sensitive to capillary perfusion and represents bulk motion of intra-vascular water protons within imaging voxels. Intravoxel incoherent motion (IVIM), a more so-phisticated approach than the conventional 2-b value approach, which describes the relationship between signal attenuation in tissues with an increasing b value, uses multiple b values (in the range of 4–10). This technique enables quantita-tive parameters that separately reflect tissue diffu-sivity and tissue microcapillary perfusion to be estimated. In principle, vascular perfusion of tumor areas can be evaluated in IVIM diffusion imaging, without the need to use gadolinium MR contrast agents. However, it is important to be aware of certain limitations of this technique, particularly the low signal-to-noise ratio in bone, which is inherently present with IVIM DWI (see **Fig. 4**). Furthermore, IVIM studies have focused primarily on brain and body imaging applications and, to the best of our knowledge, there is scant litera-ture on the application of this technique to bone lesions. Although these limitations present many challenges, IVIM may provide complementary in-formation to ADC and standardized uptake value

(SUV) in PET/MR imaging, thus warranting further attention.

Investigation of PET/MR using [18F]fluoride shows great promise in detecting bone metasta-ses caused by prostate cancer. PET/MR will allow the evaluation of several quantitative imag-ing biomarkers of disease activity and treatment response, such as the maximum SUV, mean ADC, IVIM, perfusion fraction, fast component of diffusion, and slow component of diffusion. This is a novel approach to address an unmet medical need and will support further clinical vali-dation of PET/MR as a novel imaging biomarker (**Fig. 9**).

BULLETED SUMMARY

- MR imaging provides excellent contrast be-tween a metastatic osseous lesion and normal, healthy fatty bone marrow.
- Whole-body rapid MR is now technically feasible and extremely accurate.
- FDG-PET/CT and MR showed extremely high sensitivities and specificities and were signifi-cantly more accurate for bone metastasis detection than bone scan and CT.

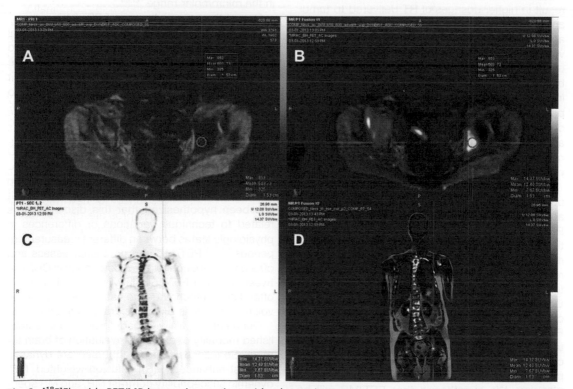

Fig. 9. [18F]Fluoride PET/MR images in a patient with advanced prostate cancer. Axial DWI (*A*) showed a low ADC (ADC = 0.3) of an intensely avid left acetabular metastases on fused PET/ADC (*B*). Coronal PET (*C*) and fused PET/T1 (*D*) show multiple osseous metastases throughout the axial skeleton.

- Although is believed MR can be more sensitive for smaller bone metastases, PET can be more specific for differentiating benign from malignant lesions, thus the potential for PET/MR to be superior than either modality individually.
- [18F]Fluoride PET/CT has been reported to have a significantly higher sensitivity compared with planar and SPECT BS for the detection of skeletal metastases in prostate cancer with high-risk for bone metastases.
- Combined PET and MR data may provide complimentary information in evaluating biological activity and treatment response of tumor, particularly using DWI.
- PET/MR will allow the evaluation of several quantitative imaging biomarkers of disease activity and treatment response, such as the maximum SUV, mean ADC, IVIM, perfusion fraction, fast component of diffusion, and slow component of diffusion.

PET/MR FOR RT PLANNING

Recent state-of-the art radiotherapy (RT) techniques, such as proton therapy and intensity-modulated RT,[45] will result in more targeted and individualized RT. This situation can theoretically result in higher dosages of RT delivered to tumor and sparing of adjacent organs. These techniques are dependent on accurate localization of tumor volume by CT.[46] Recently, PET/CT has been used to more accurately target treatment using biological tumor volume. Furthermore, molecular imaging is being explored to target radiosensitive parts of neoplasms.[47] The current thinking is that combining the biological data of PET with the anatomic correlation of CT allows for more accurate tumor delineation and radiation therapy planning.

MR offers superior tumor delineation to CT, particularly in the brain, head/neck, pelvic, and musculoskeletal primary tumors. Moreover, PET/MR data are acquired simultaneously, potentially allowing for more accurate anatomic and metabolic coregistration and minimizing patient/respiratory motion artifact. There are several potential RT applications with non-FDG-PET tracers. One future potential RT application may include contouring meningiomas with [68Ga]DOTATOC PET/MR.[48] Similarly, there is ongoing research using [11C]choline for prostate cancer detection,[49] carbon 11-PET/MR may provide more precise prostate target volume delineation for radiation planning. We hypothesize that PET/MR will be an important imaging modality of future RT planning.

NEUROLOGIC APPLICATIONS

Hybrid PET/MR is a promising new imaging modality for neurologic disease processes. The merging of these 2 modalities allows for synergy between the metabolic data of PET with the superb anatomic resolution of MR. In addition, this modality would provide increased convenience for patients who may have a baseline brain MR and PET/CT, particularly for evaluation of seizure and dementia. PET/MR has the potential to decrease radiation dose; this could be particularly helpful for the pediatric populations.

MR is superior to other radiographic examinations, with its higher soft tissue contrast, excellent structural evaluation, and millimetric spatial resolution. Brain MR has greater specificity in disease evaluation and is also the gold standard in evaluation of small intracranial structures. MR also has the ability to assess small changes in soft tissue as well as additional biological parameters.[50–52]

The strength of PET lies in continually advancing ability to evaluate functional processes and biochemical and molecular markers. However, PET suffers from limited spatial resolution, which is one of the strong points of MR. Quantitative biological values on PET can be measured in the pico-molar range, whereas MR provides high resolution in the micromolar range.[53,54]

One of the potential areas of PET/MR research will likely be in cerebral perfusion and cerebral blood flow (CBF) for the evaluation of stroke and ischemia. MR and PET/CT both have quantitative techniques to measure these processes, albeit MR is more commonly used. MR techniques to measure CBF include arterial spin labeling, dynamic susceptibility contrast imaging, and blood oxygen level–dependent MR.[52,55,56]

Some examples of PET tracers include $H_2^{15}O$ tracers, which are considered the gold standard for measuring CBF. There is a discrepancy in CBF quantitative values between PET and MR. It has been hypothesized that this discrepancy is related to technique variations or differences in physiologic states between different measurement periods.[57–59] PET/MR can potentially assess and offer an explanation for the discrepancy in CBF between MR and PET. Similarly, both PET and MR offer different techniques to assess cerebral blood volume as well as oxygen extraction fraction.

Quantitative MR with gadolinium is the established modality of choice in evaluation of brain tumors. Sequences that can be used are dynamic contrast-enhanced MR, diffusion-weighted MR, dynamic susceptibility contrast MR, and MR spectroscopy.[60] One of the well-known limitations of MR is that contrast enhancement of the brain is linked to an intact blood-brain barrier. Once the blood-brain barrier is breached, the usefulness of MR in assessment of brain tumors is significantly decreased. Factors such as CBF, cerebral blood volume, permeability, and surface area of the capillary bed are also integral components for the enhancement of brain tumors on dynamic contrast-enhanced MR. These kinetics tend to be severely altered after therapy, which explains why MR is limited in assessment of evaluating recurrence or residual neoplasm.[61]

Certain PET tracers are useful in assessment of brain tumors and can circumvent some of the MR limitations. The tracers that can be used in the evaluation of brain tumors are FDG (glucose metabolism), [11C]methionine and [18F]fluoroethyltyrosine (amino acid transport), [18F]fluorothymidine (cellular proliferation), and [18F]fluoromisonidazole (tissue hypoxia).[62,63] Given the ongoing challenges of treating several brain tumors, there is a strong need for additional imaging modalities that could aid in early diagnosis and more targeted treatment of brain malignancies. There is much research into biochemical markers targeting angiogenesis and cytotoxicity,[64] and it is likely that PET/MR would be a robust imaging tool in such research studies, allowing the investigator to examine early metabolic changes in addition to the anatomic details of MR.

Moreover, it is difficult to differentiate posttreatment radiation changes from residual tumor on MR, because posttreatment scarring/fibrosis complicates anatomic assessment and lowers specificity.[65] This is an area in which PET/MR will excel, because PET can more specifically detect recurrence in brain tumors after radiation.[65] Moreover, PET is more sensitive than anatomic imaging to assess response to treatment and is unaffected by the blood-brain barrier. Although high physiologic uptake can limit FDG cerebral PET value, there is much ongoing research with newer PET tracers.

Neurodegenerative disorders such as Alzheimer dementia (AD) affect a large percentage of the aging population.[66] The dementia spectrum includes several different dementias with distinct clinical features and treatments. The diagnosis of the correct dementia subtype is imperative to aid referring physicians in patient management and to avoid mistreatment.

Although MR has been more recently used to exclude other diseases in the workup of dementia, there are also evolving volumetric assessments of hippocampal or entorhinal cortex atrophy used to diagnose AD.[67] There are other research techniques for differentiating dementia subtypes, including MR spectroscopy and functional MR.[68]

In addition, MR has research-based techniques for dementia that allow assessment of functional processes such as diffusion tensor imaging, functional MR, and quantitative MR morphology. However, these techniques have not been proved to be highly sensitive or specific.[69,70]

On the contrary, PET tracers have been extensively studied and used in the clinical evaluation of dementia disorders. FDG-PET/CT shows a high sensitivity and specificity. These tracers range from measuring the metabolism of glucose levels to assessment of different neurotransmitters in the brain (dopamine, serotonin, and cholinergic) and evaluation of β-amyloid plaques in the brain.[71,72] Although there is much interest in amyloid plaque imaging, researchers still do not understand the relationship between CBF, structural changes on MR, and amyloid plaques. PET/MR would provide the ideal hybrid imaging modality for further understanding of this relationship in the pathogenesis of AD.

Furthermore, simultaneous PET/MR will likely minimize patient motion and misregistration of separately acquired PET and MR data, which is imperative for correlating glucose metabolism/blood flow to subtle cerebral anatomic areas.

Another evolving area of research in which PET/MR could offer diagnostic usefulness is the area of mixed dementias; current literature defines mixed dementias as AD with vascular disease, AD with vascular risk factors, or AD with any other dementing illness (such as Lewy body dementia).[73] Moreover, some literature suggests that the prevalence of mixed dementia is vastly underreported and discovered only at autopsy.[74] This theory has significant clinical implications, because misdiagnosis of a specific dementia pattern in a patient with mixed dementia may expose patients to unnecessary treatment cost and side effects, without significant effect on behavior and functional status.[75] In our early clinical experience, we have seen multiple diseases detected on PET/MR that would not have been detected on solely PET/CT or MR, thus showing the additional value of hybrid PET/MR (**Fig. 10**).

Epilepsy is another area in which PET/MR could be of clinical usefulness. MR is an important component of the workup in a patient with epilepsy. It is essential for structural lesion detection as well as the preoperative surgical planning of resection of a seizure focus.[76] The clinical usefulness of PET in epilepsy lies in the ability to detect an interictal focus of hypometabolism, commonly in the mesial temporal lobes. PET is often used when the MR is normal or discordant from other examinations such as electroencephalography. Moreover, when there is more than 1 structural

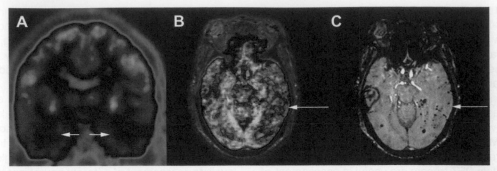

Fig. 10. A 71-year-old man for evaluation of dementia presents with PET (*A*) temporal and parietal gray matter hypometabolism typical of AD, left greater than right (*short arrows*). Overlay of simultaneously acquired PET and susceptibility-weighted imaging (SWI) (*B*) and SWI (*C*) shows susceptibility artifacts (*long arrow*, small hypointense foci), in keeping with amyloid angiopathy in addition to AD.

abnormality on the MR image, PET can be helpful in distinguishing the culprit lesion.[77,78] The combination of PET/MR may also decrease the need for ictal/interictal SPECT examinations. Because molecular changes often precede structural changes, PET/MR holds future potential for epilepsy imaging.

SUMMARY

- PET/MR can combine 2 imaging studies and provide increased convenience for patients who require a baseline brain MR and PET/CT, particularly for evaluation of seizure and dementia.
- Brain MR is superior to other radiographic examinations, with a higher soft tissue contrast, excellent structural evaluation, and millimetric spatial resolution.
- MR is the gold standard in evaluation of small intracranial structures.
- Potential areas of PET/MR research will likely be in cerebral perfusion and CBF for the evaluation of stroke and ischemia, combining the abilities of PET and MR to measure quantitative cerebral processes.
- MR can be limited in assessment of evaluating recurrence or residual neoplasm after surgery/RT; PET can more specifically detect recurrence in brain tumors after radiation.[65]
- The strength of PET/MR will lie in the evaluation of patients with dementia because both modalities provide complementary information and allow for diagnosis of mixed dementias and superimposed diseases.

LIMITATIONS

As with any new technology, there are ongoing limitations with PET/MR. One of the most crucial

steps will be the further improvement of attenuation correction of PET/MR images, thus allowing for accurate reconstructed images and calculations of SUV. Current applied T1-weighted Dixon-based attenuation correction sequences do not provide bone attenuation correction values. This limitation originates from the lack of cortical bone signal on conventional MR sequences and makes bone segmentation suboptimal in attenuation maps derived from such sequences.[79] Ongoing research is being conducted to resolve this issue by using ultrashort echo time sequences, which allow the visualization of bones (**Fig. 11**).

Other topics of concern include limited MR spatial resolution in detection of small lung nodules, compared with CT. However, more recent literature has suggested that specific MR sequences can detect subcentimetric lung nodules with high accuracy; the sensitivity of a half-Fourier acquisition single-shot turbo spin echo sequence for detecting known pulmonary nodules was 85.4%. More specifically, the sensitivity for nodules is 100%, 95.7%, 86.3%, and 73% for nodules greater than 10 mm, 6 to 10 mm, 3 to 5 mm, and smaller than 3 mm, respectively.[80] New MR sequences with improved sensitivity for lung nodule detection are under development.

RADIATION RISK

There has been increasing awareness of the detrimental effects of ionizing radiation among the general public. To ensure the best level of imaging care, it is imperative that the medical imaging community makes every effort toward the lowest possible radiation exposure. PET/CT administers approximately 25 mSv of radiation exposure,[81] whereas the CT portion accounts for half of the total radiation. The significantly lower radiation

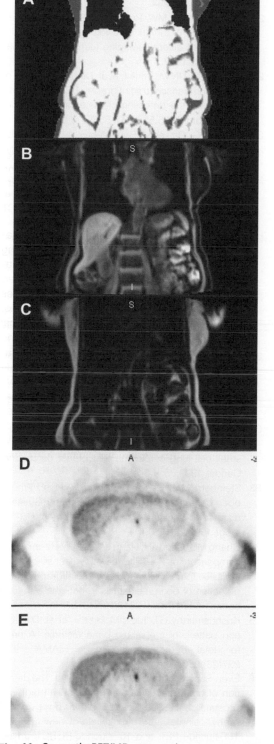

Fig. 11. Currently PET/MR attenuation maps are produced from an approximately 20-second breath-hold T1-weighted Dixon gradient echo sequence (*A*, coronal u map; *B*, coronal Dixon water image; *C*, coronal Dixon fat image; *D*, axial PET without attenuation correction; *E*, axial PET with attenuation correction).

exposure from PET/MR is a crucial advantage in its future development in oncology and neurology applications, in particular for pediatric patients.

SUMMARY

Simultaneous PET/MR is a promising novel technology for oncology diagnosis and staging and neurologic and cardiac applications. Our institution's current research protocol results in a total imaging time of approximately 45 to 70 minutes with simultaneous PET/MR imaging, making this a feasible total body imaging protocol. Further development of MR-based attenuation correction will improve PET quantification. Quantitatively accurate multiparametric PET/MR data sets will likely improve diagnosis of disease and help guide and monitor the therapies for individualized patient care.

REFERENCES

1. Jemal A, Siegel R, Ward E, et al. Cancer statistics. CA Cancer J Clin 2007;2007(57):43–66.
2. Pfister DG, Johnson DH, Azzoli CG, et al. American Society of Clinical Oncology treatment of unresectable non-small-cell lung cancer guideline: update 2003. J Clin Oncol 2004;22:330–53.
3. Knoepp UW, Ravenel JG. CT and PET imaging in non-small cell lung cancer. Crit Rev Oncol Hematol 2006;58:15–30.
4. Steinert HC. PET and PET-CT of lung cancer. Methods Mol Biol 2011;727:33–51.
5. Williams DE, Pariolero PC, Davis CS, et al. Survival of patients surgically treated for stage I lung cancer. J Thorac Cardiovasc Surg 1981;82:70–6.
6. Akata S, Kajiwara N, Park J, et al. Evaluation of chest wall invasion by lung cancer using respiratory dynamic MR. J Med Imaging Radiat Oncol 2008;52:36–9.
7. Plathow C, Aschoff P, Lichy MP, et al. Positron emission tomography/computed tomography and whole-body magnetic resonance imaging in staging of advanced non-small cell lung cancer: initial results. Invest Radiol 2008;43(5):290–7.
8. Both M, Schultze J, Reuter M, et al. Fast T1- and T2-weighted pulmonary MR-imaging in patients with bronchial carcinoma. Eur J Radiol 2005; 53(3):478–88.
9. Schwenzer N, Schrami C, Muller M. Pulmonary lesion assessment: comparison of whole-body hybrid MR/PET and PET/CT imaging–pilot study. Radiology 2012;264:2.
10. Scott W, Gobar L, Terry J, et al. Mediastinal lymph node staging of non-small-cell lung cancer: a prospective comparison of computed tomography

and positron emission tomography. J Thorac Cardiovasc Surg 1996;111:642–8.

11. Weng E, Tran L, Rege S, et al. Accuracy and clinical impact of mediastinal lymph node staging with FDG-PET imaging in potentially resectable lung cancer. Am J Clin Oncol 2000;23:47–52.

12. Kim YN, Yi CA, Lee KS, et al. A proposal for combined MRI and PET/CT interpretation criteria for preoperative nodal staging in non-small-cell lung cancer. Eur Radiol 2012;22:1537–46.

13. Mittman C, Bruderman I. Lung cancer: to operate or not? Am Rev Respir Dis 1977;116:1477–96.

14. Englemen RM, McNamara WL. Bronchogenic carcinoma: a statistical review of two hundred and thirty-four autopsies. J Thorac Surg 1954;27: 227–37.

15. Honigschnabl S, Gallo S, Niederle B, et al. How accurate is MR imaging in characterisation of adrenal masses: update of a long-term study. Eur J Radiol 2002;41(2):113–22.

16. Wu TH, Huang YH, Lee JJ, et al. Radiation exposure during transmission measurements: comparison between CT- and germanium-based techniques with a current PET scanner. Eur J Nucl Med Mol Imaging 2004;31:38–43.

17. Takahara T, Imai Y, Yamashita T, et al. Diffusion weighted whole body imaging with background body signal suppression (DWIBS): technical improvement using free breathing, STIR and high resolution 3D display. Radiat Med 2004;22:275–82.

18. Holzapfel K, Duetsch S, Fauser C, et al. Value of diffusion weighted MR imaging in the differentiation between benign and malignant cervical lymph nodes. Eur J Radiol 2009;72:381.

19. Canto MI, Hruban RH, Fishman EK, et al. Frequent detection of pancreatic lesions in asymptomatic high-risk individuals. Gastroenterology 2012; 142(4):796–804.

20. Belião S, Ferreira A, Vierasu I, et al. MR imaging versus PET/CT for evaluation of pancreatic lesions. Eur J Radiol 2012;81(10):2527–32.

21. Sahani D, Kalva S, Fischman A, et al. Detection of liver metastases from adenocarcinoma of the colon and pancreas: comparison of mangafodipir trisodium–enhanced liver MR and whole-body FDG-PET. Am J Roentgenol 2005;185(1):239–46.

22. Loeffelbein DJ, Souvatzoglou M, Wankerl V, et al. PET-MRI fusion in head-and-neck oncology: current status and implications for hybrid PET/MRI. J Oral Maxillofac Surg 2012;70(2):473–83.

23. Nishioka T, Shiga T, Shirato H, et al. Image fusion between 18FDG-PET and MRI/CT for radiotherapy planning of oropharyngeal and nasopharyngeal carcinomas. Int J Radiat Oncol Biol Phys 2002; 53:1051.

24. King AD, Tse GM, Yuen EH, et al. Comparison of CT and MR imaging for the detection of extranodal neoplastic spread in metastatic neck nodes. Eur J Radiol 2004;52:264.

25. van den Brekel MW, Runne RW, Smeele LE, et al. Assessment of tumour invasion into the mandible: the value of different imaging techniques. Eur Radiol 1998;8:1552.

26. Ghanem N, Uhl M, Brink I, et al. Diagnostic value of MRI in comparison to scintigraphy, PET, MS-CT and PET/CT for the detection of metastases of bone. Eur J Radiol 2005;55(1):41–55.

27. Schmidt G, Reiser M, Baur-Melnyk A. Whole-body imaging of bone marrow. Semin Musculoskelet Radiol 2009;13:120–33.

28. Buhmann-Kirchhoff SB, Becker C, Duerr HR, et al. Detection of osseous metastases of the spine: comparison of high resolution multi-detector-CT with MR. Eur J Radiol 2009;69(3):567–73.

29. Yang HL, Liu T, Wang XM, et al. Diagnosis of bone metastases: a meta-analysis comparing 18FDG PET, CT, MRI and bone scintigraphy. Eur Radiol 2011;21:2604–17.

30. Schmidt GP, Schoenberg SO, Schmid R, et al. Screening for bone metastases: whole-body MRI using a 32-channel system versus dual-modality PET-CT. Eur Radiol 2007;17(4):939–49.

31. Altehoefer C, Ghanem N, Hogerle S, et al. Comparative detectability of bone metastases and impact on therapy of magnetic resonance imaging and bone scintigraphy in patients with breast cancer. Eur J Radiol 2001;40:16–23.

32. Layer G, Steudel A, Schuller H, et al. MRI to detect bone marrow metastases in the initial staging of small cell lung carcinoma and breast carcinoma. Cancer 1999;85:1004–9.

33. Steinborn MM, Heuck AF, Tiling R, et al. Whole-body bone marrow MRI in patients with metastatic disease to skeletal system. J Comput Assist Tomogr 1999;23:123–9.

34. Chang MC, Chen JH, Liang JA, et al. Meta-analysis: comparison of F-18 fluoro-deoxyglucose-positron emission tomography and bone scintigraphy in the detection of bone metastasis in patients with lung cancer. Acad Radiol 2012;19:349–57.

35. Krishnamurthy GT, Tubis M, Hiss J, et al. Distribution pattern of metastatic bone disease. A need for total body skeletal image. JAMA 1977; 237(23):2504–6.

36. Even-Sapir E, Metser U, Mishani E, et al. The detection of bone metastases in patients with high-risk prostate cancer: 99mTc-MDP planar bone scintigraphy, single- and multi-field-of-view SPECT, 18F-fluoride PET, and 18F-fluoride PET/CT. J Nucl Med 2006;47(2):287–97.

37. Yeh SD, Imbriaco M, Larson SM, et al. Detection of bony metastases of androgen-independent prostate cancer by PET-FDG. Nucl Med Biol 1996;23: 693–7.

38. Cook GJ, Fogelman I. The role of positron emission tomography in skeletal disease. Semin Nucl Med 2001;31:50–61.

39. Fogelman I, Cook G, Israel O, et al. Positron emission tomography and bone metastases. Semin Nucl Med 2005;35:135–42.

40. Schiepers C, Nuytes J, Bormans G, et al. Fluoride kinetics of the axial skeleton measured in vivo with fluorine-18-fluoride PET. J Nucl Med 1997;38:1970–6.

41. Israel O, Goldberg A, Nachtigal A, et al. FDG-PET and CT patterns of bone metastases and their relationship to previously administered anti-cancer therapy. Eur J Nucl Med Mol Imaging 2006;33(11):1280–4.

42. Mosavi F, Johansson S, Sandberg DT, et al. Whole-body diffusion-weighted MRI compared with 18F-NaF PET/CT for detection of bone metastases in patients with high-risk prostate carcinoma. Am J Roentgenol 2012;199(5):1114–20.

43. Fizazi K, Albiges L, Massard C, et al. Novel and bone-targeted agents for CRPC. Ann Oncol 2012;23(Suppl 10):264–7.

44. Reischauer C, Froehlich JM, Koh DM, et al. Bone metastases from prostate cancer: assessing treatment response by using diffusion-weighted imaging and functional diffusion maps–initial observations. Radiology 2010;257:523–31.

45. Muzik J, Soukup M, Alber M. Comparison of fixed-beam IMRT, helical tomotherapy, and IMPT for selected cases. Med Phys 2008;35:1580–92.

46. Rit S, Nijkamp J, van Herk M, et al. Comparative study of respiratory motion correction techniques in cone-beam computed tomography. Radiother Oncol 2011;100:356–9.

47. van der Heide UA, Houweling AC, Groenendaal G, et al. Functional MRI for radiotherapy dose painting. Magn Reson Imaging 2012;30:1216–23.

48. Gehler B, Paulsen F, Oksuz MO, et al. [68 Ga]-DOTATOC-PET/CT for meningioma IMRT treatment planning. Radiat Oncol 2009;4:56.

49. Van den Bergh L, Koole M, Isebaert S, et al. Is there an additional value of 11C-choline PET-CT to T2-weighted MRI images in the localization of intraprostatic tumor nodules? Int J Radiat Oncol Biol Phys 2012;83:1486–92.

50. Werner MK, Schmidt H, Schwenzer NF. MR/PET: a new challenge in hybrid imaging. AJR Am J Roentgenol 2012;199(2):272–7.

51. Catana C, Cherry S, Sorensen A. Combined positron emission tomography and magnetic resonance imaging scanners–potential neurological applications. Neuroradiology 2008;4(2):76–80.

52. Balyasnikova S, Löfgren J, de Nijs R, et al. PET/MR in oncology: an introduction with focus on MR and future perspectives for hybrid imaging. Am J Nucl Med Mol Imaging 2012;2(4):458–74.

53. Daftary A. PET-MRI: challenges and new directions. Indian J Nucl Med 2010;25(1):3–5.

54. Heiss W. The potential of PET/MRI for brain imaging. Eur J Nucl Med 2009;36(Suppl 1):105–12.

55. Catana C, Drzezga A, Heiss W, et al. PET/MRI for neurologic applications. J Nucl Med 2012;53:1916–25.

56. Donahue MJ, Lu H, Jones CK, et al. An account of the discrepancy between MRI and PET cerebral blood flow measures. A high-field MRI investigation. NMR Biomed 2006;19(8):1043–54.

57. Heiss WD, Sobesky J. Comparison of PET and DW/PW-MRI in acute ischemic stroke. Keio J Med 2008;57(3):125–31.

58. Heiss WD. Ischemic penumbra: evidence from functional imaging in man. J Cereb Blood Flow Metab 2000;20(9):1276–93.

59. Carroll TJ, Teneggi V, Jobin M, et al. Absolute quantification of cerebral blood flow with magnetic resonance, reproducibility of the method, and comparison with H2(15)O positron emission tomography. Cereb Blood Flow Metab 2002;22(9):1149–56.

60. Fink JR, Carr RB, Matsusue E, et al. Comparison of 3 Tesla proton MR spectroscopy, MR perfusion and MR diffusion for distinguishing glioma recurrence from posttreatment effects. J Magn Reson Imaging 2012;35(1):56–63. http://dx.doi.org/10.1002/jmri.22801.

61. Chassidim Y, Vekslor R, Lublinsky S, et al. Quantitative imaging assessment of blood-brain barrier permeability in humans. Fluids Barriers CNS 2013;10(1):9.

62. Chen W. Clinical applications of PET in brain tumors. J Nucl Med 2007;48(9):1468–81.

63. Herholz K, Langen KJ, Schiepers C, et al. Brain tumors. Semin Nucl Med 2012;42(6):356–70. http://dx.doi.org/10.1053/j.semnuclmed.2012.06.001.

64. Jain RK, di Tomaso E, Duda DG, et al. Angiogenesis in brain tumours. Nat Rev Neurosci 2007;8(8):610–22.

65. Ricci PE, Karis JP, Heiserman JE, et al. Differentiating recurrent tumor from radiation necrosis: time for re-evaluation of positron emission tomography? AJNR Am J Neuroradiol 1998;19(3):407–13.

66. Mazziotta JC, Frackowiak RS, Phelps ME. The use of positron emission tomography in the clinical-assessment of dementia. Semin Nucl Med 1992;22(4):233–46.

67. Chetelat G, Landeau B, Eustache F, et al. Using voxel-based morphometry to map the structural changes associated with rapid conversion in MCI: a longitudinal MRI study. Neuroimage 2005;27(4):934–46.

68. Kantarci K. H-1 Magnetic resonance spectroscopy in dementia. Br J Radiol 2007;80:S146–52.

69. Health Quality Ontario. Functional brain imaging: an evidence-based analysis. Ont Health Technol Assess Ser 2006;6(22):1–79.

70. Sheline YI, Raichle ME. Resting state functional connectivity in preclinical Alzheimer's disease. Biol Psychiatry 2013;74(5):340–7.

71. Le bars D. Fluorine-18 and medical imaging: radiopharmaceuticals for positron emission tomography. J Fluor Chem 2006;127:1488–93.

72. Drzezga A, Lautenschlager N, Siebner H, et al. Cerebral metabolic changes accompanying conversion of mild cognitive impairment into Alzheimer's disease: a PET follow-up study. Eur J Nucl Med Mol Imaging 2003;30:1104–13.

73. Zekry D, Hauw JJ, Gold G. Mixed dementia: epidemiology, diagnosis and treatment. J Am Geriatr Soc 2002;50:1431–8.

74. Jellinger KA. Alzheimer disease and cerebrovascular pathology: an update. J Neural Transm 2002; 109:813–36.

75. Kavirajan H, Schneider LS. Efficacy and adverse effects of cholinesterase inhibitors and memantine in vascular dementia: a meta-analysis of randomised controlled trials. Lancet Neurol 2007;6: 782–92.

76. Won HJ, Chang KH, Cheon JE, et al. Comparison of MR imaging with PET and ictal SPECT in 118 patients with intractable epilepsy. AJNR Am J Neuroradiol 1999;20(4):593–9.

77. Singhal T. Positron emission tomography applications in clinical neurology. Semin Neurol 2012; 32(4):421–31.

78. Widjaja E, Li B, Medina LS. Diagnostic evaluation in patients with intractable epilepsy and normal findings on MRI: a decision analysis and cost-effectiveness study. AJNR Am J Neuroradiol 2013;34(5):1004–9.

79. Samarin A, Burger C, Wollenweber SD, et al. PET/MR imaging of bone lesions–implications for PET quantification from imperfect attenuation correction. Eur J Nucl Med Mol Imaging 2012;39(7):1154–60.

80. Schroeder T, Ruehm SG, Debatin JF, et al. Detection of pulmonary nodules using a 2D HASTE MR sequence: comparison with MDCT. AJR Am J Roentgenol 2005;185:979–84.

81. DeGrado TR, Turkington TG, Williams JJ, et al. Performance characteristics of a whole-body PET scanner. J Nucl Med 1994;35:1398–406.

Index

Note: Page numbers of article titles are in **boldface** type.

A

Abdomen
 FDG-PET/CT imaging for, **169–183**
  artifacts in, 178
  benign conditions in, 178–180
  brown adipose tissue and, 176–177
  medication effects of, 176–177
  patient preparation for, 174–175
  physiologic activity, 170–174
  skeletal muscle and, 178
 FDG-PET/MR imaging for, 240–241
Abscesses
 abdominal, 178–179
 liver, 179–180
Actinomycosis, of chest wall, 155
Acute respiratory distress syndrome, 158
Adenomas, hepatic, 179–180
Adenomyosis, uterine, 190–191
Adipose tissue. See also Brown adipose tissue.
 of thorax, FDG uptake in, 148
Adnexal benign pathology, 191
Adrenal glands, FDG-PET/CT imaging for, 173–174,
 210–215, 230
Advantages Workstation, 121
Age factors, in FDG-PET/CT imaging, 132–134
Alcohol, FDG-PET/CT imaging effects of, 134–135
Alzheimer disease, hypometabolism in, 134
Amphetamines, FDG-PET/CT imaging effects of, 135
Amyloidosis, of thorax, 165
Anesthesia
 FDG-PET/CT imaging effects of, 136
 for pediatric imaging, 198–199, 202
Anus, FDG-PET/CT imaging for, after radiotherapy,
 225–226
Aorta, disorders of, 164
Appendicitis, 187–188
Artifacts, in FDG-PET/CT imaging
 of abdomen, 178
 of brain, 136–137
 of head and neck, 145
Asbestosis, 158
Aspiration pneumonia, 155–156
Atherosclerosis
 iliac vessel, 188
 myocardial, 163–164
Atrium, FDG uptake in, 163
Atropine, for colon preparation, 175
Attenuation calculation, in FDG-PET/CT imaging, 137

B

Background activity clearance, of FDG, 209–215
Barrett esophagus, 164
Benner tumors, 191
Benzodiazepines, in FDG-PET/CT imaging
 effects of, 136
 in pediatric patients, 198–199
 of thorax, 158
Berylliosis, 158
Bezafibrate, in FDG-PET/CT imaging, of thorax,
 158
Biliary tract, FDG-PET/CT imaging for, 179–180
Biological errors, in FDG-PET/CT quantification, 124
Biopsy, in thorax, 160
Bladder catheterization, in pediatric patients, 202,
 206–207
Bladder, FDG-PET/CT imaging for, 170–172,
 174–175
 after radiotherapy, 227–228
 in benign pathology, 188
Bone, metastasis to, FDG-PET/MR imaging for,
 243
Bone marrow, FDG-PET/CT imaging for
 after radiotherapy, 230–231
 FDG uptake in, 148–149, 204
 medication effects on, 177
 of abdomen, 177
 of thorax, 148–149
Brachytherapy, 232
Brain
 FDG-PET/CT imaging for, **129–140**
  after radiotherapy, 218–220
  age factors in, 132–134
  artifacts in, 136–137
  gender differences in, 134
  in pediatric patients, 196–197, 200–204
  medications and substances affecting,
   134–136
  normal anatomy in, 130–131
  radiotherapy effects on, 136
  scanning time for, 131–132
  technique for, 130
 FDG-PET/MR imaging for, 246–248
Breast, FDG uptake in, 148
Brown adipose tissue, FDG uptake in
 in pediatric patients, 198–199
 of abdomen, 176–177
 of thorax, 148

PET Clin 9 (2014) 253–257
http://dx.doi.org/10.1016/S1556-8598(14)00011-X
1556-8598/14/$ – see front matter © 2014 Elsevier Inc. All rights reserved.

C

Caffeine, FDG-PET/CT imaging effects of, 134
Cancer staging
    FDG-PET/CT for, quantification of
        errors in, 122–124
        in clinical trials, 124
        personnel qualification in, 121–122
        quality control in, 120–121
        standardization in, 120
        SUV measurement in, 118–120
    FDG-PET/MR imaging for, **237–252**
        clinical applications for, 240–248
        principles of, 238
        results reporting in, 238–239
        technique for, 238
Cardiac implantable electronic device, infections
    of, 56
Catheter-insertion sites, in thorax, 160
Cecum, FDG-PET/CT imaging for, 170
Chemotherapy, FDG-PET/CT imaging with, 136,
    158
Chest. See Thorax.
Chest wall, infections of, 155
Chronic obstructive pulmonary disease, 149–150
Churg-Strauss syndrome, 158
Clinical trials, in FDG-PET/CT quantification, 124
Coal-related lung disease, 158
Cocaine, FDG-PET/CT imaging effects of, 135–136
Colitis, 170
Colon, FDG-PET/CT imaging for, 170–172, 174–177,
    186–188
Connective tissue disease, interstitial lung disease in,
    158
Contrast agents, for abdominal imaging preparation,
    175
Contusions, chest, 162–163
Corticosteroids, FDG-PET/CT imaging effects of,
    136
Crohn's disease, 170, 180
Cystic fibrosis, 162

D

Defibrillator insertion, 160
Dementia, hypometabolism in, 134
Dermatomyositis, interstitial lung disease in, 158
Diabetes mellitus, FDG-PET/CT imaging with, 198
Diphenoxylate, for colon preparation, 174–175
Distraction techniques, for pediatric imaging, 202
Distribution time, of FDG, 209–215
Diverticula
    bladder, 188
    esophageal, 170, 180
    tracheal, 164
Diverticulitis, 187
Drainage tubes, in chest, 160

E

Elastofibroma dorsi, in subscapular region, 164–165
Elderly persons, FDG-PET/CT imaging for, in brain,
    133–134
Endocarditis, infectious, 156
Endometriomas, 191
Endometriosis, 190–191
EORTC (European Organization for Research and
    Treatment of Cancer) criteria, 119, 121
Errors, in FDG-PET/CT quantification, 122–124
Esophagitis, 222–223
Esophagus, FDG-PET/CT imaging for
    after radiotherapy, 222–223
    FDG uptake in, 155, 205
    in benign disorders, 164
European Organization for Research and Treatment
    of Cancer (EORTC) criteria, 119, 121

F

Fallopian tubes, FDG uptake in, 206
Fasting, in pediatric patient preparation, 196–198
FDG-PET/CT imaging
    abdomen, **169–183**
    brain. See Brain.
    differential background clearance, **209–216**
    for malignant disease staging, **117–127**
    head and neck, **141–145**
    pediatric, **195–208**
    pelvis, **185–193**
    postradiation changes, **217–235**
    thorax, **146–168**
FDG-PET/MR imaging, **237–252**
    clinical applications for, 240–248
    limitations of, 248
    principles of, 238
    radiation risks in, 248–249
    results reporting in, 238–239
    technique for, 238
Fentanyl, in FDG-PET/CT imaging, 198–199
Fibromas, adnexal, 191
Fibrothecomas, 191
Fibrous dysplasia, pelvic, 186
[18F]-Fluorodeoxyglucose. See FDG.
Focal nodular hyperplasia, 179–180
Fractures, 149, 186
Furosemide, for bladder preparation, 174–175

G

Gallbladder, polyps of, 180
Gastrointestinal tract, FDG-PET/CT imaging for
    after radiotherapy, 222–226
    FDG uptake in, 155, 205
    in benign conditions, 178–180
    medication effects of, 176–177

of chest, 155
    patient preparation for, 174–175
    physiologic activity, 170–172
Gender differences, in FDG-PET/CT imaging, 134
Genitourinary tract, FDG-PET/CT imaging for
    after radiotherapy, 226–228
    FDG uptake in, 206–207
    in benign conditions, 180
    patient preparation for, 174–175
    physiologic activity, 171–173
Granulocyte colony-stimulating factor, in FDG-PET/
    CT imaging, 158

H

Hamartomas
    pulmonary, 162
    tracheal, 164
Head and neck
    FDG-PET/CT imaging for, **141–145**
        artifacts in, 145
        benign findings in, 144
        interpretation of, 142
        physiologic FDG uptake and, 142–144
        protocol for, 141–142
    FDG-PET/MR imaging for, 241–242
Heart. See also Myocardium.
    contusions of, 162–163
    FDG uptake in, 151–155, 204
Hematomas, abdominal, 178–179
Hemothorax, 162–163
Hepatocellular carcinoma, 179–180
Hyperglycemia, in FDG-PET/CT imaging, 136–137,
    198
Hypometabolism, in brain, 134

I

Iliac vessels, FDG-PET/CT imaging for, 188
Infections
    adnexal, 191
    chest wall, 155–157
Infectious endocarditis, 156
Inflammatory bowel disease, 170, 180
Intellectual disabilities, management issues with, 202
Interstitial lung disease, 157–158
Intrauterine contraceptive devices, 191
Intubation, tracheal stenosis in, 164
Kidney, FDG-PET/CT imaging for, 171, 180, 226–227

L

Larynx, FDG uptake in, 143–144, 204
Leiomyomas
    esophageal, 164
    tracheal, 164
    uterine, 190
Leiomyosarcomas, uterine, 190

Leydig cells, FDG-PET/CT imaging for, 189
Lipomas, tracheal, 164
Lipomatous hypertrophy, of atrial septum, 163
Liver, FDG-PET/CT imaging for, 173, 179–180
    after radiotherapy, 228–229
    FDG clearance in, 210–215
    in benign conditions, 179–180
Lung
    cancer of, 239–240
    contusions of, 162–163
    FDG-PET/CT imaging for, 239–240
        FDG clearance in, 210–215
        FDG uptake in, 150
    FDG-PET/MR imaging for, 239–240
    interstitial disease of, 157–158
    transplantation of, 160–161
Lymph nodes, FDG uptake in
    FDG clearance in, 210–215
    of chest, 155
    of head and neck, 144
Lymphatic tissue, FDG uptake in, 204

M

Magnetic resonance imaging, in FDG-PET/MR
    imaging, **237–252**
Mediastinal blood pool
    FDG clearance in, 210–215
    FDG uptake in, 148, 151–152
Mediastinal infections, 156
Mediastinoscopy, 160
Medications, in FDG-PET/CT imaging
    of brain, 134–136
    of gastrointestinal tract, 176–177
    of thorax, 158
Menstrual cycle, FDG uptake and, 189, 206
Metal prostheses, artifacts due to, 178
Metastasis, FDG-PET/MR imaging for, 240–241
Metformin, in FDG-PET/CT imaging
    for pediatric patients, 198
    of gastrointestinal tract, 176–177, 186–187
    of thorax, 158
Microscopic polyangiitis, 158
Motion artifacts, in FDG-PET/CT imaging
    of abdomen, 178
    of brain, 137
Muscles, FDG uptake in
    abdominal, 178
    clearance of, 210–215
    head and neck, 143
    in pediatric patients, 199–200, 206–207
    thoracic, 149–150
Myocarditis, 156–158, 204
Myocardium
    disorders of, 163–164
    FDG clearance in, 210–215
    FDG uptake in, 151–155, 204

N

Neck. *See* Head and neck.
Nephropathy, radiation, 226–228
Neurogenic tumors, tracheal, 164
Neuroleptic drugs, FDG-PET/CT imaging effects of, 136
Nodules, pulmonary, 162

O

Oncocytomas, 180
Osteoarthritis, pelvic, 186
Osteomyelitis, of chest wall, 155
Osteoradionecrosis, 230–231
Ovary, FDG-PET/CT imaging for, 189–191, 206

P

Pacemaker insertion, 160
Paget disease, pelvic, 186
Pancreas, FDG-PET/CT imaging for, 173
    after radiotherapy, 229
    FDG clearance in, 210–215
    in benign conditions, 180
Pancreatitis, 180
Papillomas, tracheal, 164
Paraspinal muscles, FDG uptake in, 149
Parotid gland, benign tumors of, 144
Pediatric patients
    FDG-PET/CT imaging for, **195–208**
        FDG uptake in, 148–149
        image coregistration in, 203
        in brain, 132–133
        in marrow, 148–149
        indications for, 203
        normal uptake patterns in, 204–207
        patient preparation for, 196–201
        protocols for, 201–202
        special concerns in, 202–203
    labeled sodium fluoride imaging for, 195
Pelvis
    FDG-PET/CT imaging for, **185–193**
    FDG-PET/MR imaging for, 240–241
PERCIST (PET Response Criteria in Solid Tumors)
    criteria, 119, 121
Pericarditis, postradiation, 158
Pericardium, FDG uptake in, 152
Personnel, qualification of, 121–122
PET Response Criteria in Solid Tumors (PERCIST)
    criteria, 119, 121
Pharyngeal muscles, FDG uptake in, 204
Physical errors, in FDG-PET/CT quantification,
    123–124
Placenta, FDG-PET/CT imaging for, 189–191
Pleomorphic adenoma, of salivary glands, 144
Pleura, FDG uptake in, 150

Pleural effusion, 160
Pleurodesis, 160
Pneumoconioses, 158
Pneumonia, 155–156
Pneumonitis, radiation, 158, 222
Pneumothorax, 162–163
Polychondritis, relapsing, of trachea, 164
Polymyositis, interstitial lung disease in, 158
Polyps
    colonic, 180, 186–187
    gallbladder, 180
Pregnancy, FDG-PET/CT imaging in, 189–191, 203
Propranol, in FDG-PET/CT imaging, in pediatric
    patients, 198–199
Prostate
    cancer of
        brachytherapy for, 232
        FDG-PET/MR imaging for, 243–246
    FDG-PET/CT imaging for, 188–189
Prosthetic heart valves, infections of, 156–157
Pulmonary fibrosis, interstitial, 157–158
Pulmonary hilar nodes, FDG uptake in, 155
Pulmonary hypertension, 164
Pulmonary nodules, 162

Q

Quality control, in PET/CT quantification, 120–121
Quantification, of cancer staging. *See* Cancer
    staging.

R

Radiation pneumonitis, 222
Radioembolization, 231–232
Radiofrequency ablation, in thorax, 158–159
Radiotherapy
    FDG-PET/CT imaging after, **217–235**
        bone and bone marrow, 230–231
        brain, 136
        central nervous system, 218–221
        external, 218–222
        gastrointestinal system, 222–226
        genitourinary system, 226–228
        injury classification of, 218
        internal, 231–232
        lung, 221–222
        prostate, 232
        solid organs, 228–230
        thorax, 158, 221–222
    planning for, FDG- PET/MR imaging for, 246
RECIST (response evaluation criteria in solid tumors)
    guidelines, for treatment response evaluation,
    119, 121
Rectum, FDG-PET/CT imaging for, after
    radiotherapy, 225–226
Relapsing polychondritis, of trachea, 164

Response evaluation criteria in solid tumors (RECIST) guidelines, for treatment response evaluation, 119, 121
Restrictive lung disease, 157–158
Retroperitoneal fibrosis, 179
Rheumatoid arthritis, interstitial lung disease in, 158
Rib, fractures of, 162–163

S

Salivary glands, FDG uptake in, 143–144, 204
Sarcoidosis, 161–162
Sedation, for pediatric imaging, 198–199, 202
Senna-glycoside, for colon preparation, 174–175
Seromas, abdominal, 179
Sertoli cells, FDG-PET/CT imaging for, 189
Silicosis, 158
Sjögren syndrome, 158
Skin, of thorax, FDG uptake in, 148
Small intestine, FDG-PET/CT imaging for, after radiotherapy, 223–225
Solid organs, FDG-PET/CT imaging for
    after radiotherapy, 228–230
    physiologic activity, 173–174
Spinal cord, FDG-PET/CT imaging for
    after radiotherapy, 220–222
    FDG uptake in, 144
Spine, fractures of, 149
Spleen, FDG-PET/CT imaging for, 173, 177
    after radiotherapy, 229
    FDG clearance in, 210–215
    FDG uptake in, 204
    medication effects on, 177
Standardization, in PET/CT quantification, 120
Standardized uptake values, in FDG-PET/CT, 118–120, 210–215
Sternotomy, 149, 160
Stomach, FDG-PET/CT imaging for
    after radiotherapy, 223–225
    FDG uptake in, 205–206
Systemic lupus erythematosus, interstitial lung disease in, 158

T

Talc pleurodesis, 160
Technical errors, in FDG-PET/CT quantification, 122–123
Teratomas, adnexal, 191
Thorax, FDG-PET/CT imaging for, **147–168**
    benign pathologic FDG uptake patterns in, 157–165
    normal FDG biodistribution patterns in, 148–155
Thrombosis
    iliac vessel, 188
    myocardial, 163–164
Thymus, FDG uptake in, 151, 153, 204
Thyroid gland, FDG uptake in, 144
Tonsils, FDG uptake in, 143
Trachea, disorders of, 164
Transplantation, lung, 160–161
Trauma, chest, 162–163
Truncation artifact, in thoracic FDG-PET/CT imaging, 148
Tuberculosis
    chest wall, 155
    pericardial, 156–157

U

Ulcerative colitis, 170, 180
Ureter, FDG-PET/CT imaging for, 171
Uterus, FDG-PET/CT imaging for, 189–191

V

Vasculitis, pulmonary, 158
Vertebroplasty, 149
Vocal cords, FDG uptake in, 143–144

W

Warthin's tumor, 144
Wegener granulomatosis, 158
Whole-body FDG-PET/CT imaging, background clearance in, 209–215

Moving?

Make sure your subscription moves with you!

To notify us of your new address, find your **Clinics Account Number** (located on your mailing label above your name), and contact customer service at:

Email: journalscustomerservice-usa@elsevier.com

800-654-2452 (subscribers in the U.S. & Canada)
314-447-8871 (subscribers outside of the U.S. & Canada)

Fax number: 314-447-8029

Elsevier Health Sciences Division
Subscription Customer Service
3251 Riverport Lane
Maryland Heights, MO 63043

*To ensure uninterrupted delivery of your subscription, please notify us at least 4 weeks in advance of move.

ELSEVIER

Printed and bound by CPI Group (UK) Ltd, Croydon, CR0 4YY

03/10/2024

01040379-0008